Challenges and Controversies in Kidney Transplantation

Challenges and Controversies in Kidney Transplantation

Editor

Sandip Kapur MD FACS

G Tom Shires, MD Faculty Scholar in Surgery

Professor of Surgery

Weill Cornell Medical College

Chief, Division of Transplant Surgery

NewYork-Presbyterian/Weill Cornell Medical Center

New York, New York, USA

Foreword

David A Gerber MD FACS

JAYPEE The Health Sciences Publisher

New Delhi | London | Philadelphia | Panama

JAYPEE **Jaypee Brothers Medical Publishers (P) Ltd**

Headquarters
Jaypee Brothers Medical Publishers (P) Ltd.
4838/24, Ansari Road, Daryaganj
New Delhi 110 002, India
Phone: +91-11-43574357
Fax: +91-11-43574314
E-mail: jaypee@jaypeebrothers.com

Overseas Offices
J.P. Medical Ltd.
83, Victoria Street, London
SW1H 0HW (UK)
Phone: +44-20 3170 8910
Fax: +44(0)20 3008 6180
E-mail: info@jpmedpub.com

Jaypee-Highlights Medical Publishers Inc.
City of Knowledge, Bld. 237, Clayton
Panama City, Panama
Phone: +1 507-301-0496
Fax: +1 507-301-0499
E-mail: cservice@jphmedical.com

Jaypee Medical Inc.
The Bourse
111, South Independence Mall East
Suite 835, Philadelphia, PA 19106, USA
Phone: +1 267-519-9789
E-mail: jpmed.us@gmail.com

Jaypee Brothers Medical Publishers (P) Ltd.
17/1-B, Babar Road, Block-B, Shaymali
Mohammadpur, Dhaka-1207
Bangladesh
Mobile: +08801912003485
E-mail: jaypeedhaka@gmail.com

Jaypee Brothers Medical Publishers (P) Ltd.
Bhotahity, Kathmandu, Nepal
Phone: +977-9741283608
E-mail: kathmandu@jaypeebrothers.com

Website: www.jaypeebrothers.com
Website: www.jaypeedigital.com

Inquiries for bulk sales may be solicited at: jaypee@jaypeebrothers.com

Challenges and Controversies in Kidney Transplantation

First Edition: **2015**

ISBN: 978-93-5152-525-7

Printed at Replika Press Pvt. Ltd.

Contributors

Meredith J Aull Pharm D
Assistant Research Professor of Surgery
Weill Cornell Medical College
Director of Clinical Research & Quality
Kidney & Pancreas Transplant Program
NewYork-Presbyterian/Weill Cornell
Medical Center
New York, New York, USA

Laurence J Belin MD MPH
Department of Surgery
NewYork-Presbyterian/Weill Cornell
Medical Center
New York, New York, USA

Sean Campbell MD
Department of Medicine
Weill Cornell Medical College
New York, New York, USA

Darshana M Dadhania MD MS
Associate Professor of Medicine
Weill Cornell Medical College
Associate Attending Physician
Assistant Director, Immunogenetics and
Transplantation Center
NewYork-Presbyterian/Weill Cornell
Medical Center
New York, New York, USA

Sandip Kapur MD FACS
G Tom Shires, MD Faculty Scholar in Surgery
Professor of Surgery
Weill Cornell Medical College
Chief, Division of Transplant Surgery
NewYork-Presbyterian/Weill Cornell
Medical Center
New York, New York, USA

Jim Kim MD
Assistant Professor of Surgery
Weill Cornell Medical College
Assistant Attending Surgeon
NewYork-Presbyterian/Weill Cornell
Medical Center
New York, New York, USA

Jennifer McDermott Pharm D BCPS
Clinical Pharmacy Manager
Solid Organ Transplantation
NewYork-Presbyterian/Weill Cornell
Medical Center
New York, New York, USA

Thangamani Muthukumar MD
Assistant Professor of Medicine
Weill Cornell Medical College
Assistant Attending Physician
NewYork-Presbyterian/Weill Cornell
Medical Center
New York, New York, USA

Pallavi Patri MD
Instructor in Medicine
Weill Cornell Medical College
Assistant Attending Physician
NewYork-Presbyterian/Weill Cornell
Medical Center
New York, New York, USA

Patricia Myers-Gurevitch MD
Department of Medicine
Weill Cornell Medical College
New York, New York, USA

Mary Simmerling PhD
Assistant Professor of
Research Integrity in Medicine
Weill Cornell Medical College
New York, New York, USA

Anthony C Watkins MD
Assistant Professor of Surgery
Weill Cornell Medical College
Assistant Attending Surgeon
NewYork-Presbyterian/Weill Cornell
Medical Center
New York, New York, USA

Foreword

In the nearly two decades since Dr Sandip Kapur and I completed our time as clinical transplant fellows at the Starzl Transplantation Institute at the University of Pittsburgh, I have watched the NewYork-Presbyterian/Weill Cornell Kidney Transplant Program flourish under Sandip's leadership. The program has cultivated an exemplary reputation by applying innovative strategies to address and overcome some of the challenges that are inherent in kidney transplantation. The NewYork-Presbyterian/Weill Cornell program has established itself as a recognized leader in several areas including: early adoption and utilization of expanded criteria deceased donor organs, a standardized immunosuppression regimen to enable early corticosteroid withdrawal, single site nephrectomy for living kidney donors, and kidney paired donation for patients with incompatible living donors.

In this textbook, Dr Kapur and his colleagues provide a thorough and clear overview of topics along two main themes: increasing the organ donor pool for patients with end stage renal disease who are in need of a renal transplant and strategies to manage the challenging transplant candidate and recipient populations. In the first section, methods to increase organ availability are discussed, including transplantation of expanded deceased donor organs such as those from older donors, pediatric donors, donors with co-morbidities, and donors with hepatitis C infection, as well as increasing access to living donor kidney transplantation through pioneering minimally invasive donor surgery and Kidney Paired Donation. The second section of the book focuses on challenging patient population at the extremes of age, patients with hepatitis C and/or HIV infection, and patients who develop post-transplant infectious or immunologic complications. The textbook closes with strategies to personalize the immunosuppression regimens of these complex patient populations.

Transplant professionals will find this textbook a useful learning tool, due to the insights offered on progress and novel advances to increase their patients' chances of receiving a kidney transplant, and on ways to successfully transplant and manage challenging patient populations.

David A Gerber MD FACS
Professor of Surgery
Chief, Abdominal Transplant Surgery
University of North Carolina School of Medicine
Chapel Hill, North Carolina, USA

Preface

Although renal transplantation is a relatively young field in medicine, with the first successful kidney transplant occurring in 1954, the past 15 years have shown rapid advances in many areas within transplantation, and the next 15 years hold great promise for further advancement. Unfortunately, the shortage of deceased donor organs continues to be the major limiting factor in transplantation, particularly as the waiting list grows in the setting of a complex and aging population. Successful transplant programs must work diligently to maximize opportunities for transplantation for their patients, including utilization of marginal donor organs, pediatric organs, and hepatitis C positive organs. By considering the use of such organs in carefully selected recipients, the organs that are available can be utilized to the greatest extent possible, with acceptable if not excellent outcomes. Development of minimally invasive techniques has advanced the field of living kidney donation, and rapid advances in kidney paired donation registries have enabled transplantation of many patients who initially presented with a willing but incompatible living donor. The first section of this book focuses on ways programs can maximize transplant opportunities for their patients.

The complex nature of transplantation requires transplant centers to manage many challenges on both a programmatic and patient level. We believe it is helpful for centers to share their experience with challenging patient populations in order to benefit the entire field. In the second section of this book, we focus on management of select patient populations, such as children, the elderly, HIV and hepatitis C positive patients, highly sensitized patients, and patients who develop post-transplant polyomavirus nephropathy. In addition, we discuss how to personalize immune regimens based on patient-specific factors. The need for tools to monitor transplant recipients and therapies to treat these patients for the complications of over-immunosuppression is an important target for research and development.

We hope that the reader finds this book to be a comprehensive resource on the topics mentioned above as well as others that can help transplant centers offer transplantation to as many candidates as possible, and improve post-transplant outcomes in order to maximize the organs that are donated.

Sandip Kapur MD FACS

Acknowledgments

Challenges and Controversies in Kidney Transplantation represents the collective effort of a talented group of professionals and support staff at the NewYork-Presbyterian/Weill Cornell Medical Center. These professionals have dedicated their careers to advancing the field of transplantation and creating the best patient experience possible. The core clinical mission of our program has been to maximize all opportunities for transplantation for the patients who seek our help. I want to thank my colleagues whose invaluable contributions have enhanced transplant opportunities for our patients and who have made this textbook a remarkable collection of chapters that describe the NewYork-Presbyterian/Weill Cornell kidney transplant experience.

I want to thank my chairman, Dr Fabrizio Michelassi for his support, guidance, and his faith in me to build a program that provides the finest in transplant care. I am also greatly appreciative of Dr David Gerber for his review and contribution in writing the foreword to this textbook. I would also like to thank the professionals at Jaypee Brothers Medical Publishers for their guidance in the preparation of this textbook.

Most important, I want to thank our patients who serve as an inspiration for all of our efforts, and I am grateful for the trust they place in us to provide their transplant care. Lastly, I want to thank my family, especially my children, who remind me each day that life is precious and invaluable.

Contents

1

SECTION

Maximizing Transplant Opportunities

Utilization of Marginal, Pediatric and HCV+ Deceased Donor Organs

CHAPTER 1

Jim Kim

ABSTRACT

The disparity between organ supply and demand continues to grow, resulting in an ever-growing need to increase the donor pool. As a result, the utilization of suboptimal or marginal donors has become a common strategy to lessen this organ shortage. Although these donors serve as valuable resources, increased rates of delayed graft function and primary nonfunction and inferior graft survival rates highlight the importance of appropriate donor selection and recipient matching. By maximizing these marginal donors, access to transplantation can be optimized without compromising outcomes.

INTRODUCTION

Extraordinary breakthroughs in the realm of transplantation have been made since the first successful kidney transplant by Joseph Murray and his team in 1954. Advancements in immunosuppressive drug therapies, enhanced understandings of immunology, and changes in public policy have all led to significantly improved outcomes over the past six decades. According to data compiled by the National Institute of Diabetes and Digestive and Kidney Diseases (NIDDK) and National Institute of Health (NIH), the 5-year patient survival rate for transplant recipients is 85.5% compared to 35.8% for dialysis patients (Fig. 1.1).[1] The landmark paper by Wolfe and colleagues in 1999 also showed a doubling of life expectancy in renal transplant patients as compared to those who were wait-listed and remained on dialysis.[2] This study demonstrated the long-term mortality (>18 months) was reduced by 68% in recipients of deceased donor renal transplants. These findings have led to an explosion in the number of patients with end-stage renal disease (ESRD) being listed for kidney transplants. What was once considered "a respite from the real treatment of dialysis"[3] is now the accepted therapeutic approach for those with kidney failure.

As of November 1, 2013, there were over 98,000 candidates listed for a kidney transplant.[4] Despite the increasing numbers of people with ESRD in need of a transplant, there has not been a concordant rise in the number of

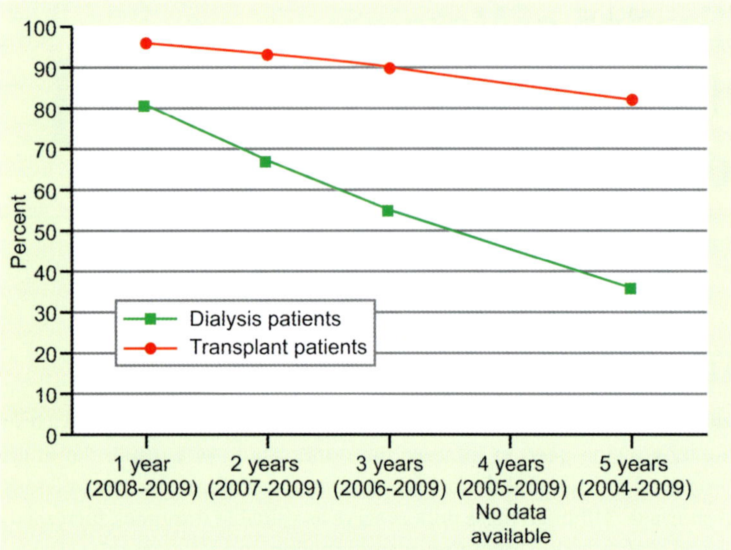

Fig. 1.1: Patient survival rates by dialysis and transplant.
Source: NIH Publication No. 12-3895 June 2012 (National Institute of Diabetes and Digestive and Kidney Diseases, National Institutes of Health).

Table 1.1: Kidney transplants by donor type in the United States.

Donor type	*2001*	*2011*
All deceased donors	8234 (100)	11,043 (100)
Standard criteria donor	7033 (85.41)	9,374 (84.89)
Expanded criteria donor (ECD)	1201 (14.59)	1,669 (15.11)
Donation after cardiac death, non-ECD	227 (2.76)	1,592 (14.42)
Donation after cardiac death, ECD	16 (0.19)	106 (0.96)

Data from 2011 OPTN & SRTR Annual Data Report.
Values expressed as number (percent).

organ donors. This has resulted in a steady decline in the rate of transplants for adult candidates on the waiting list. The rate of deceased donor renal transplants performed in 1998 was 20.6 transplants per 100 wait-list years as compared to 11.4 transplants per 100 wait-list years in 2011.[5] With this growing disparity between supply and demand, there is an imperative to expand the pool of donors. One strategy is to use organs previously thought to be unacceptable (Table 1.1). A growing body of evidence has shown promising results using kidney allografts from marginal and pediatric donors, as well as from donors with hepatitis C.[4,6-8] Despite inferior outcomes compared to standard criteria donors (SCD), these donors may help to alleviate the organ shortage because the negative impact of dialysis is far worse than the negative impact of "inferior" grafts. Key factors in successful utilization of these donors include selecting appropriate donor traits, weighing recipient characteristics and managing variable risk factors to optimize outcomes.

MARGINAL DONORS

Expanded Criteria Donor

Donor Criteria and Outcomes

An analysis of the Scientific Registry of Transplant Recipients (SRTR) was undertaken to study "expanded" qualities of donors.[9] A consensus definition for expanded criteria donors (ECDs) was developed to describe basic characteristics that were associated with a 70% greater likelihood of graft loss [relative risk (RR) >1.7] as compared to SCD.[6,10] These factors included age and three statistically significant risk factors: history of arterial hypertension, cause of death from cerebrovascular accident, and preretrieval serum creatinine >1.5 mg/dL. Consequently, ECD was implemented as policy starting October 31, 2002 and was defined as donor age over 60 or over age 50 plus any 2 of the 3 cited risk factors.[11]

A landmark paper by Ojo et al. associated certain clinical features, which included advanced age, long-standing hypertension, diabetes mellitus, and prolonged cold ischemic time (CIT), with inferior outcomes compared to ideal kidney donors.[12] However, the authors determined a substantial survival advantage using these 'marginal' donors over those wait-listed patients maintained on dialysis, showing an average increase of 5 years in life expectancy. Prior to this study, no accepted definition of a "marginal" donor had existed and the SRTR study soon afterwards defined ECD to standardize this type of kidney.

In another important study, Merion et al. demonstrated the adjusted risk of death at 3 years for recipients of an ECD kidney was 60% lower than for wait-listed transplant candidates.[13] For non-ECD transplants, the mortality reduction was even greater at 72%. Overall, the relative long-term mortality was found to be 17% lower for ECD recipients than those who had standard therapy (wait-listed for transplant, maintained on dialysis or receiving SCD).

The long-term graft outcomes of ECD may be worse in comparison to SCD, but the overall mortality is significantly reduced compared with those remaining on dialysis.[14] ECD was shown to have similar early graft survival compared to SCD, but this was shown to be significantly less after a mean follow-up of 50 months. Regardless, using ECD kidneys was still found to be more cost-effective than maintenance on dialysis.[15] An earlier study by Stratta et al. determined that the estimated half-lives of ECD kidneys were 6–8 years compared to 10–12 years in SCD kidneys,[16] and both far exceeded established patient survival on dialysis. The adjusted patient survival for

Table 1.2: Recipient characteristics for ECD kidneys.[13,17]

Beneficial	*Disadvantageous*
Age >40 years	Age <40 years
Diabetes or hypertension as cause of ESRD	Short waiting time
Listed in OPO with long waiting time (>1350 days)	Retransplantation
Non-hispanic	

OPO, organ procurement organizations

ECD as compared to non-ECD at 1 and 5 years was found to be 90.6% and 69% vs 94.5% and 81.2%, respectively.[10] The overall patient survival for those remaining on dialysis at 5 years was <40%.[1]

Optimizing Outcomes

To achieve the maximum benefit from ECD, it becomes increasingly important to identify the best possible setting in which to use these donors (Table 1.2). No standard protocol has been established, but several studies have highlighted the significance of appropriate donor selection to match recipient characteristics. There are considerable differences across organ procurement organizations (OPOs) in the proportion of candidates wait-listed for ECD.[18] In OPOs where median waiting times are prolonged (>1350 days), the risk of death was 27% lower for ECD recipients. However, in OPOs where wait times were shorter, an ECD survival benefit was only shown for diabetic recipients. In addition, a subgroup, consisting of patients over age 40 years, those with hypertension or diabetes, non-Hispanics, and unsensitized patients, were shown to have significant survival benefit with ECD kidney transplants.[13] Older recipients have been shown to be good candidates for ECD kidneys because graft survival typically exceeds patient survival on dialysis. Patients over age 60 years who were recipients of ECD kidneys had a 62% greater death rate at 1 year than recipients of SCD, but had a significant survival advantage over patients remaining on dialysis.[19] Another study demonstrated increased survival in recipients over the age of 60 years receiving kidneys from donors over the age of 70 years as compared to recipients aged 41–60 years.[20] For patients over age 40 years, the benefits conferred by an SCD kidney were negated by the additional years on dialysis. There appeared to be no upper age limit; even patients exceeding age 75 years attained a survival benefit. For diabetics aged 18–39 years, receiving kidneys from ECD after 2 years had a similar life expectancy compared to those waiting 4 years for SCD.[21] However, cumulative survival of ECD recipients did not equilibrate with patients waiting for a transplant until 3.5 years posttransplantation due to the excess ECD recipient mortality.[13]

One of the most common indications for transplantation is failure of an existing allograft.[22] Although repeat kidney transplantation has been shown to improve patient survival over dialysis therapy, using ECD kidneys may not be a cost-effective strategy[23] because retransplantation with ECD kidneys has poor outcomes. This subgroup of patients likely has better outcomes remaining on dialysis until an SCD or living donor become available.[17] A review of the SRTR database demonstrated a 56% decrease in mortality with repeat transplants using SCD. However, similar survival was found between those remaining on the waiting list compared to repeat transplant with ECD.[24]

Stroke as the cause of death in the donor also portends a worse outcome, with inferior graft half-life, patient survival, and a RR of 2.2 for graft loss.[6,25,26] ECDs have also been associated with increased urinary complications, but did not result in increased graft loss.[27] ECDs were also noted to have higher rates of delayed graft function (DGF), primary nonfunction (PNF), and lower creatinine clearance at 5 years. However, in comparing ECD to SCD, 5-year graft (70.4% vs 76.7%) and patient survival (88.2% vs 88.9%) were not significantly different.[28]

Especially because of intrinsic disease and loss of nephron mass that occurs with normal aging, careful selection of ECD is important to successful outcomes. In fact, over 50% of all procured kidneys that were discarded were from ECD.[5] Perioperative mortality risk for ECD kidney transplantation has been shown to be 5.2-fold higher within the first 2 weeks compared to standard therapy. This risk decreases and only becomes equal at 33 weeks post-transplant.[13] Several factors determine whether ECD would be suitable to use for transplant. Donor creatinine clearance (CrCl) can serve as a surrogate for projected kidney function from single or dual kidney (both kidneys from same donor) transplants. Single kidneys were used with a CrCl >65 mL/min, dual kidneys were used for CrCl 40–65 mL/min, and kidneys were discarded if CrCl was <40 mL/min.[16] The use of donor biopsies are controversial, but can also potentially be a useful tool in selecting appropriate ECD kidneys. Glomerulosclerosis >20% has been identified to be a risk factor for early graft failure.[29] Remuzzi et al. devised a scoring system centered on histological evaluation prior to kidney allocation.[30] This study suggested similar outcomes using dual ECD kidneys compared to SCD based on four histological factors: glomerulosclerosis, arteriosclerosis, tubular atrophy, and interstitial fibrosis (Table 1.3). The current UNOS (United Network of Organ Sharing) guidelines considers dual kidney allocation if any two of the following criteria exist: donor age >60 years, estimated donor CrCl <65 mL/min, rising serum creatinine (>2.5 mg/dL) at time of procurement, donor history of long-standing hypertension or diabetes mellitus, or adverse donor kidney histology (defined as glomerulosclerosis of 15–50%).

Another strategy to improve outcomes with ECD is to limit the CIT, which appears to have a more deleterious effect than for SCD.[12,16,31] The

Table 1.3: Pretransplant biopsy factors and allocation of dual kidney transplant.[30]

	0	1+	2+	3+
Glomerulosclerosis	None	<20%	20–50%	>50%
Tubular atrophy	Absent	<20%	20–50%	>50%
Interstitial fibrosis	Absent	<20%	20–50%	>50%
Arterial/arteriolar narrowing	Absent	<Luminal diameter	≥Luminal diameter	Extreme narrowing or occlusion
Total score	0–3 (mild)	4–6 (moderate)		7–12 (severe)
Use for transplant	Single kidney	Dual kidney		Discard kidneys

prevalence of DGF, which has been associated with impaired long-term graft survival,[12,32,33] can be partly attributed to the increased sensitivity of ECD to the effects of cold ischemia.[34] However, the impact of CIT has also been called into question in a recent analysis of the SRTR database. Despite DGF rates being higher for CIT >15 h and significantly more likely between pairs with greater CIT (35% vs 31%, P <0.001), graft and patient survival were similar.[35] The authors noted no association with acute rejection. A safe conclusion from these conflicting studies would be to minimize CIT when possible, but it is not advisable to automatically discard ECD solely based on prolonged CIT. Minimizing CIT also relates to how these kidneys are stored. Although multiple studies have evaluated the effects of static cold storage (CS) and pulsatile machine perfusion (MP), their individual merits can be debatable.[36,37] In regards to ECD, there appears to be a significant reduction in DGF using MP over CS.[37–39] The long-term patient and graft survival rates do not seem markedly improved, but still appear to be a cost-effective strategy.[40,41]

Donation After Cardiac Death

Since the criteria for brain death was defined in 1968, most transplants have resulted from donation after brain death (DBD).[42] However, rates of donation after cardiac death (DCD) have increased from 1.4% in 1998 to 15.8% in 2011.[5] In other countries, such as Japan, DCD comprises the majority of organ donors. Unlike in brain dead donors, organs from DCD donors are procured after cardiopulmonary arrest and face warm ischemic injury until cold preservation solution is perfused. Concerns about poor graft function arose due to this additional ischemic insult, especially with higher rates of DGF and PNF being reported.[43] However, follow-up studies over the past two decades demonstrate similar long-term patient and graft survival compared to DBD donors.[44] Increasing numbers of DCD organs can contribute to expansion of the donor pool and help alleviate the shortage of organs.

Despite a higher incidence of DGF and PNF, these complications do not appear to have a negative effect on long-term outcomes.[45] One large study from the University of Wisconsin demonstrated higher rates of DGF and discharge creatinine with the use of DCD kidneys, but no difference was found in long-term graft survival. DBD renal transplants had a 5-, 10-, and 15-year graft survival of 71.3%, 48.3%, and 33.8%, while DCD renal transplants had graft survival of 64.8%, 44.8%, and 27.8%, respectively.[46] In another study, 45% of DCD renal transplants experienced DGF, but that had no effect on graft and patient survival or kidney function.[47] This study also suggested that increased donor age was associated with higher risk of poor kidney function with the highest observed risk being donors older than 45 years (RR 4.81, p=0.001). Other clinical features, such as CIT >12 hour, have also been shown to increase rates of DGF in kidney transplants using DCD donors. However, both DCD and DBD donors under age 50 years old had similar graft survival.[48]

Attention to clinical features also impact successful outcomes for DCD donors. Warm ischemia time, donor age, length of CIT, and method of preservation have been studied and optimizing these variables can lead to liberal use of kidneys from these donors.[49] Techniques, such as mechanical chest compression devices and extracorporeal membrane oxygenation, have been suggested to help reduce the effects of warm ischemic time.[50] Contradicting studies regarding the potential benefits of MP over CS have been reported.[36,51] Overall, MP appears to reduce DGF, but its implication to long-term graft survival remains controversial.[52] As previously cited, multiple studies have also shown donor age to be correlated with DGF. An analysis of the SRTR database demonstrated ECD status did not adversely affect the outcomes of DCD kidney transplant (hazard ratio 1.04; 95% CI, 1.01–1.15) compared to non-ECD (hazard ratio 1.21; 95% CI, 1.04–1.40). The study suggested ECD-DCD donor kidneys could be a valuable source of potential donors.[53] At the other end of the age spectrum, kidneys from pediatric DCD donors (aged 2–17) had similar patient and graft survival compared to their DBD counterparts.[54] Multiple studies support the conclusion that DCD kidneys can safely be utilized to expand the donor pool without detrimental consequences and can even be allocated in a similar fashion to DBD kidneys.

PEDIATRIC DONORS

The donor pool can potentially be further expanded with the use of pediatric donors for adult recipients. Much like ECD and DCD, proper matching of donor and recipient characteristics is important for good outcomes, but the optimal use of small pediatric donors has not been clearly determined.[55-57]

Suboptimal graft survival rates and higher technical complications have historically contributed to lower utilization rates from these donors, particularly from smaller pediatric donors (age <5 years, weight <20 kg). These organs have been among the highest discarded group. The use of en bloc kidneys, in part, was developed to offset some of these negative consequences, as well as to augment renal size.[58] However, transplanting solitary kidneys from these donors would maximize their use and could serve as a valuable resource to combat the organ shortage. Determining the proper situation whether to use solitary or en bloc pediatric kidneys has not been clearly elucidated.

Graft survival of en bloc pediatric donor allografts has been shown to have similar outcomes compared with adult donors.[59,60] A major concern, though, was the perceived increased graft loss associated with solitary pediatric kidneys. One analysis of the SRTR database demonstrated a 78% increased risk of graft loss for single kidneys from pediatric donors who weighed <21 kg.[56] This risk of early graft loss was theorized to be as a result of the hyperfiltration syndrome, a condition where a donor-recipient size mismatch leads to compensatory changes of hypertension, proteinuria, glomerulosclerosis and, ultimately, inadequate filtration ability.[61] Pediatric donor kidneys, though, have also been shown to increase in size and hypertrophy to provide adequate nephron mass to meet adult metabolic requirements.[57,62,63]

Other studies, however, have demonstrated comparable outcomes using solitary pediatric kidneys. For donors <5 years old, solitary pediatric kidneys were found to have a 2-year graft survival rate of 92.5% as compared to 89.8% for SCD.[64] Better 2-year actuarial graft survival rates for solitary pediatric donors of 93% have also been demonstrated compared to 77% after en bloc transplantation.[65] Another analysis of the SRTR database demonstrated solitary pediatric kidneys from donors >35 kg had similar graft survival to SCD.[66] Outcomes from adult donors between ages 18 and 45 years were found to be equivalent to grafts from these solitary pediatric donors. Actuarial death-censored graft survival at 1 year and 5 years from adult vs pediatric donors was 93% and 85% vs 93% and 84%.[67]

Mounting evidence shows the efficacy in utilizing pediatric donors for adult recipients. Attention to meticulous surgical technique and proper patient selection can result in excellent long-term outcomes. Despite conflicting data with respect to the superiority of en bloc kidneys, selective use of solitary pediatric kidneys can clearly be justified. Current data suggest donor age likely serves as a surrogate marker for the size of the kidneys. Further studies looking at specific donor and recipient characteristics need to be conducted, but pediatric kidneys can safely be used as solitary kidneys when donors weigh >15 kg and are >6 cm in length.

HEPATITIS C POSITIVE DONORS

Approximately 3.2 million people in the United States are infected with hepatitis C virus (HCV).[68] Compared to HCV(-) patients, HCV(+) patients wait-listed for kidney transplantation have a higher risk of death than HCV(-) patients.[69] HCV(+) status has also been shown to be an independent risk factor for death and graft loss after kidney transplant.[70] However, a significant survival benefit is seen after transplant for HCV(+) recipients compared to those who remain on dialysis.[71] Due to their increased rates of morbidity and mortality, it becomes more important to expand the donor pool to make more organs available. HCV(+) patients are a unique population of patients wait-listed for a kidney transplant who can benefit from HCV(+) donors.

For appropriate patients, the use of HCV(+) donors can potentially expand the donor pool and shorten waiting times. The wait-list time for an HCV(+) patient was, on average, 395 days less than for those who were HCV(-). However, only 29% of these patients received kidneys from HCV(+) donors and HCV(+) kidneys had a 2.6 times higher rate of discard than HCV(-) kidneys.[8] Most centers will limit the use of HCV(+) donors to recipients with a positive viral load and with the most common genotype 1b. Those patients, who have cleared the virus or have less virulent genotypes, risk activation of viral replication. Poor survival was seen in HCV(-) elderly patients receiving HCV(+) kidneys due to rapid development of HCV infection, liver disease, and infectious complications.[72] Even HCV(-) recipients on the waiting list deemed to have poor life expectancy on dialysis had poor patient and graft survival when transplanted with HCV(+) kidneys. In addition, HCV(+) donor status was a negative risk factor for patient survival.[73] Regardless of recipient HCV status, an analysis of the SRTR database demonstrated poor patient survival when HCV(+) donor kidneys were utilized and only HCV(+) recipients had worse graft survival.[74] Overall patient and graft survival for HCV(+) recipients was lower compared to HCV(-) recipients, but the survival rates at 3 years between HCV(+) and HCV(-) donors were similar.[8] Despite inferior outcomes in comparison to HCV(-) patients, kidney transplantation confers a survival benefit over remaining on dialysis.[70]

ASSESSING RISK

Not all kidneys within a specific subgroup are the same. The designation for the type of kidney, i.e. SCD vs ECD, is based on a binary (yes/no) indicator and has been used to assess risk of graft failure. Due to the wide variability within these subgroups (e.g. high risk SCD vs low risk ECD), more recent studies have looked at incorporating specific donor factors in a continuous scoring system. The Kidney Donor Risk Index (KDRI) was developed to assess the RR of graft failure based on 10 donor characteristics in comparison to reference deceased donors at the median, 50th percentile from the previous year. A higher KDRI value corresponds to a higher risk of graft failure compared to an "average" donor.[75] Among the various factors, the KDRI includes donor age (pediatric vs SCD vs ECD) as well as HCV status (Table 1.4). Woodside et al. analyzed the SRTR database for utilization and outcomes for kidneys designated as ECD. Because the terms ECD and SCD do not account for donor quality within each category, higher discard rates were seen for biopsied kidneys. Although overall graft survival of ECD was worse than SCD, no difference was seen within specific KDRI intervals. The authors concluded that the ECD designation conferred no increased risk of graft failure beyond that predicted by KDRI.[76] To simplify the risk assessment, the Kidney Donor Profile Index (KDPI) converts the KDRI from a RR scale to a cumulative percentage scale. In other words, a higher KDPI confers a greater risk of graft failure. For example, a donor with a KDPI of 90% can be interpreted as being a low-quality donor because it has a KDRI >89% and at most 90% of donors in the chosen reference population.[77] In March 2012, the OPTN began including the KDPI in DonorNet℠ along with the SCD and ECD designations, but has not yet used it as a tool for allocating kidneys. Eventually, though, the OPTN Kidney Committee plans to use KDPI for "longevity matching"-attempting to minimize life years lost following death with a functioning graft while maximizing the number of life years gained with each utilized organ.[78]

Table 1.4: KDRI donor factors age (in years)

Donor characteristics	*Applies to*	*Model coefficients*
	All donors	0.0128
	Age <18	–0.0194
	Age >50	0.0107
Height (cm)	All donors	–0.0464
Weight (kg)	Weight <80 kg	–0.0199
Ethnicity	African American donors	0.1790
History of hypertension	Hypertensive donors	0.1260
History of diabetes	Diabetic donors	0.0881
Cause of death (COD)	Cerebrovascular accident	0.0881
Serum creatinine (mg/dL)	All donors	0.2200
	Creatinine >1.5	–0.2090
HCV status	HCV(+) donors	0.2400
DCD status	DCD donors	0.1330

KDRI, Kidney Donor Risk Index; HCV, hepatitis C virus; DCD, donation after cardiac death

CONCLUSION

The growth of the waiting list continues to outpace the number of available donors, and severely limits the number of patients from receiving the benefits of transplantation. Kidneys from ECD, DCD, pediatric, and HCV(+) donors have been a valuable resource in trying to offset the disparity between supply and demand. Studies have shown good outcomes from these donors, especially when carefully selected based on a variety of characteristics and limiting negative factors such as cold ischemia time. Over the past decade, the number of transplants from ECD has tripled and has increased nearly 10-fold from DCD donors. The lack of available organs continues to challenge the transplant community, but expansion of the donor pool can help to alleviate the shortage while maintaining efficacy.

REFERENCES

1. US Kidney Disease Statistics, National Kidney and Urologic Diseases Information Clearinghouse; http://kidney.niddk.nih.gov
2. Wolfe RA, Ashby VB, Milford EL, et al. Comparison of mortality in all patients on dialysis, patients on dialysis awaiting transplantation, and recipients of a first cadaveric transplant. New Engl J Med. 1999;341:1725-30.
3. Rennie D. Home dialysis and the costs of uremia. N Engl J Med. 1978;298:399-400.
4. OPTN data, US Department of Health and Human Services; http://optn.transplant.hrsa.gov
5. Matas AJ, Smith JM, Skeans MA, et al. OPTN/SRTR 2011 Annual Data Report: Kidney. Am J Transplant. 2013;13(S1):11-46.
6. Port FK, Bragg JL, Metzger RA, et al. Donor characteristics associated with reduced graft survival: an approach to expanding the pool of kidney donors. Transplantation. 2002;74(9):1281-6.
7. Pelletier SJ, Guidinger MK, Merion RM, et al. Recovery and utilization of deceased donor kidneys from small pediatric donors. Am J Transplant. 2006;6(7):1646-52.
8. Kucirka LM, Singer AL, Ros RL, et al. Underutilization of hepatitis C-positive kidneys for hepatitis C-positive recipients. Am J Transplant. 2010;10(5):1238-46.
9. Rosengard BR, Feng S, Alfrey EJ, et al. Report of the crystal city meeting to maximize the use of organs recovered from the cadaver donor. Am J Transplant. 2002;2(8):701-11.
10. Metzger RA, Delmonico FL, Feng S, et al. Expanded criteria donors for kidney transplantation. Am J Transplant. 2003;3(S4):114-25.
11. UNOS Policy 3.5.l. Expanded criteria donor definition and point system. Richmond, VA: United Network for Organ Sharing; 2002.
12. Ojo AO, Hanson JA, Meier-Kriesche H-U, et al. Survival in recipients of marginal cadaveric donor kidneys compared with other recipients and wait-listed transplant candidates. J Am Soc Nephrol. 2001;12(3):589-97.
13. Merion RM, Ashby VB, Wolfe RA. Deceased-donor characteristics and the survival benefit of kidney transplantation. JAMA. 2005;294(21):2726-33.
14. Pascual J, Zamora J, Pirsch J. A systematic review of kidney transplantation from expanded criteria donors. Am J Kidney Dis. 2008;52(3):553-86.

15. Saidi RF, Elias N, Kawai T, et al. Outcome of kidney transplantation using expanded criteria donors and donation after cardiac death kidneys: realities and costs. Am J Transplant. 2007;7(12):2769-74.
16. Stratta RJ, Rohr MS, Sundberg AK, et al. Intermediate-term outcomes with expanded criteria donors in kidney transplantation. Ann Surg. 2006;243(5): 594-603.
17. Rao PS, Schaubel DE, Wei G, et al. Evaluating the survival benefit of kidney retransplantation. Transplantation. 2006;82(5):669-74.
18. Sung RS, Guidinger MK, Leichtman AB, et al. Impact of the expanded criteria donor allocation system on candidates for and recipients of expanded criteria donor kidneys. Transplantation. 2007;84(9):1138-44.
19. Kauffman HM, McBride MA, Cors CS, Roza AM, Wynn JJ. Early mortality rates in older kidney recipients with comorbid risk factors. Transplantation. 2007; 83(4):404-10.
20. Chavalitdhamrong D, Gill J, Takemoto S. Patient and graft outcomes from deceased kidney donors age 70 years and older: an analysis of the Organ Procurement Transplant Network/United Network of Organ Sharing database. Transplantation. 2008;85(11):1573-9.
21. Schold JD, Meier-Kriesche HU. Which renal transplant candidates should accept marginal kidneys in exchange for a shorter waiting time on dialysis? Clin J Am Soc Nephrol. 2006;1(3):532-8.
22. Cohen DJ, St. Martin L, Christensen LL, Bloom RD, Sung RS. Kidney and pancreas transplantation in the United States, 1995–2004. Am J Transplant. 2006;6(5):1153-69.
23. Sellers MT, Velidedeoglu E, Bloom RD, et al. Expanded-criteria donor kidneys: a single-center clinical and short-term financial analysis - cause for concern in retransplantation. Transplantation. 2004;78(11):1670-5.
24. Miles CD, Schaubel DE, Jia X, et al. Mortality experience in recipients undergoing repeat transplantation with expanded criteria donor and non-ECD deceased donor kidneys. Am J Transplant. 2007;7(5):1140-7.
25. Matas AJ, Gillingham K, Payne WD, et al. Should I accept this kidney? Clin Transplant. 2000;14(1):90-5.
26. Johnston O, O'Kelly P, Spencer S, et al. The impact of donor spontaneous intracranial haemorrhage vs other donors on long-term renal graft and patient survival. Clin Transplant. 2006;20(1):91-5.
27. Ratner LE, Kraus E, Magnuson T, Bender JS. Transplantation of kidneys from expanded criteria donors. Surgery. 1996;119(4):372-7.
28. Dahmane D, Audard V, Hiesse C, et al. Retrospective follow-up of transplantation of kidneys from 'marginal' donors. Kidney Int. 2006;69(3):546-52.
29. Cicciarelli J, Cho Y, Mateo R, et al. Renal biopsy donor group: the influence of glomerulosclerosis on transplant outcomes. Transplant Proc. 2005;37(2):712-13.
30. Remuzzi, G, Grinyo J, Ruggenenti P, et al. Early experience with dual kidney transplantation in adults using expanded donor criteria. Double Kidney Transplant Group (DKG). J Am Soc Nephrol. 1999;10(12):2591-8.
31. Mikhalski D, Wissing KM, Ghisdal L, et al. Cold ischemia is a major determinant of acute rejection and renal graft survival in the modern era of immunosuppression. Transplantation. 2008;85(Suppl):S3-9.
32. Shoskes DA, Cecka JM. Deleterious effects of delayed graft function in cadaveric renal transplant recipients independent of acute rejection. Transplantation. 1998;66(12):1697-1701.

33. Doshi MD, Garg N, Reese PP, et al. Recipient risk factors associated with delayed graft function: a paired kidney analysis. Transplantation. 2011;91(6):666-71.
34. Johnston TD, Thacker LR, Jeon H, Lucas BA, Ranjan D. Sensitivity of expanded-criteria donor kidneys to cold ischaemia time. Clin Transplant. 2004;18(S12): S28-S32.
35. Kayler LK, Magliocca J, Zendejas I, et al. Impact of cold ischemia time on graft survival among ECD transplant recipients: a paired kidney analysis. Am J Transplant. 2011;11(12):2647-56.
36. Watson CJE, Wells AC, Roberts RJ, et al. Cold machine perfusion versus static cold storage of kidneys donated after cardiac death: a UK multicenter randomized controlled trial. Am J Transplant. 2010;10(9):1991-9.
37. Moers C, Smits JM, Maathuis M-HJ, et al. Machine perfusion or cold storage in deceased-donor kidney transplantation. New Engl J Med. 2009;360(1):7-19.
38. Matsuoka L, Shah T, Aswad S, et al. Pulsatile perfusion reduces the incidence of delayed graft function in expanded criteria donor kidney transplantation. Am J Transplant. 2006;6(6):1473-8.
39. Stratta RJ, Moore PS, Farney AC, et al. Influence of pulsatile perfusion preservation on outcomes in kidney transplantation from expanded criteria donors. J Am Coll Surg. 2007;204(5):873-82.
40. Schold JD, Kaplan B, Howard RJ, et al. Are we frozen in time? Analysis of the utilization and efficacy of pulsatile perfusion in renal transplantation. Am J Transplant. 2005;5(7):1681-8.
41. Buchanan PM, Lentine KL, Burroughs TE, et al. Association of lower costs of pulsatile machine perfusion in renal transplantation from expanded criteria donors. Am J Transplant. 2008;8(11):2391-2401.
42. Ad Hoc Committee of the Harvard Medical School to Examine the Definition of Brain Death. A definition of irreversible coma: report of the Ad Hoc Committee of the Harvard Medical School to Examine the Definition of Brain Death. JAMA. 1968;205(6):337-40.
43. Weber M, Dindo D, Demartines N, et al. Kidney transplantation from donors without a heartbeat. New Engl J Med. 2002;247(4):248-55.
44. Ledinh H, Bonvoisin C, Weekers L, et al. Results of kidney transplantation from donors after cardiac death. Transplant Proc. 2010;42(7):2407-14.
45. Singh RP, Farney AC, Rogers J, et al. Kidney transplantation from donation after cardiac death donors: lack of impact of delayed graft function on post-transplant outcomes. Clin Transplant. 2011;25(2):255-64.
46. Cooper JT, Chin LT, Krieger NR, et al. Donation after cardiac death: The University of Wisconsin experience with renal transplantation. Am J Transplant. 2004; 4(9):1490-4.
47. Wadei HM, Heckman MG, Rawal B, et al. Comparison of kidney function between donation after cardiac death and donation after brain death kidney transplantation. Transplantation. 2013;96(3):274-81.
48. Locke JE, Segev DL, Warren DS, et al. Outcomes of kidneys from donors after cardiac death: implications for allocation and preservation. Am J Transplant. 2007;7(7):1797-1807.
49. Hoogland ER, Snoeijs MG, Habets MA, et al. Improvements in kidney transplantation from donors after cardiac death. Clin Transplant. 2013;27:E295-E301.
50. Hoogland ER, Snoeijs MG, van Heurn LW. DCD kidney transplantation: results and measures to improve outcome. Curr Opin Organ Transplant. 2010;15(2): 177-82.

51. Jochman I, Mohan S, Moers C, et al. Machine perfusion versus cold storage for the preservation of kidneys donated after cardiac death. Ann Surg. 2010; 252(5):756-64.
52. Bathini V, McGregor T, McAlister VC, et al. Renal perfusion pump versus cold storage for donation after cardiac death kidneys: a Systematic Review. J Urol. 2013;189(6):2214-20.
53. Singh SK, Kim SJ. Does expanded criteria donor status modify the outcomes of kidney transplantation from donors after cardiac death? Am J Transplant. 2013;13(2):329-36.
54. de Vries EE, Snoeijs MG, van Heurn E. Kidney donation from children after cardiac death. Crit Care Med. 2010;38(1):249-53.
55. Bresnahan BA, McBride MA, Cherikh WS, et al. Risk factors for renal allograft survival from pediatric cadaver donors: an analysis of Untied Network of Organ Sharing data. Transplantation. 2001;72(2):256-61.
56. Pelletier SJ, Guidinger MK, Merion RM, et al. Recovery and utilization of deceased donor kidneys from small pediatric donors. Am J Transplant. 2006;6(7):1646-52.
57. Merkel FK. Five and 10 year follow-up of en bloc small pediatric kidneys in adult recipients. Transplant Proc. 2001;33(1-2):1168-9.
58. Dharnidharka VR, Stevens G, Howard RJ. En-bloc kidney transplantation in the United States: An analysis of the United Network of Organ Sharing (UNOS) data from 1987 to 2003. Am J Transplant. 2005;5(6):1513-7.
59. Sharma A, Fisher RA, Cotterell AH, et al. En bloc kidney transplantation from pediatric donors: comparable outcomes with living donor kidney transplantation. Transplantation. 2011;92(5):564-9.
60. Sureshkumar KK, Reddy CS, Nghiem DD et al. Superiority of pediatric en bloc renal allografts over living donor kidneys: a long-term functional study. Transplantation. 2006;82(3):348-53.
61. Mohanka R, Basu A, Shapiro R, et al. Single versus en bloc kidney transplantation from pediatric donors less than or equal to 15 kg. Transplantation. 2008;86(2): 264-8.
62. Uemura R, Liang J, Khan A, et al. Outcomes of transplantation of single pediatric renal allografts equal to or more than 6 cm in length. Transplantation. 2010;89(6):710-13.
63. Sibler SJ. Renal transplantation between adults and children differences in renal growth. JAMA. 1974;228(9):1143.
64. Balachandran VP, Aull MJ, Goris M, et al. Successful transplantation of single kidneys from pediatric donors weighing less than or equal to 10 kg into standard weight adult recipients. Transplantation. 2010;90(5):518-22.
65. Borboroglu PG, Foster III CE, Philosophe B, et al. Solitary renal allografts from pediatric cadaver donors less than 2 years of age transplanted into adult recipients. Transplantation. 2004;77(5):698-702.
66. Kayler LK, Zendejas I, Gregg A, et al. Kidney transplantation from small pediatric donors. Transplantation. 2012;96(4):430-6.
67. Csapo Z, Knight RJ, Podder H, et al. Long-term outcomes of single paediatric vs ideal adult renal allograft transplants in adult recipients. Clin Transplant. 2006;20(4):423-6.
68. Centers for Disease Control and Prevention, http://www.cdc.gov
69. Bloom RD, Sayer G, Fa K, et al. Outcome of hepatitis C virus-infected kidney transplant candidates who remain on the waiting list. Am J Transplant. 2005;5(1):139-44.

70. Fabrizi F, Martin P, Dixit V, et al. Hepatitis C virus antibody status and survival after renal transplantation: meta-analysis of observational studies. Am J Transplant. 2005;5(6):1452-61.
71. Ingasith A, Kamanamool N, Thakkinstian A, et al. Survival advantage of kidney transplantation over dialysis in patients with hepatitis C: a systematic review and meta-analysis. Transplantation. 2013;95(7):943-8.
72. Flohr TR, Bonatti H, Hranjec T, et al. Elderly recipients of hepatitis C positive renal allografts can quickly develop live disease. J Surg Res. 2012;176(2):629-38.
73. Singh N, Neidlinger N, Djamali A, et al. The impact of hepatitis C virus donor and recipient status on long-term outcomes: university of Wisconsin experience. Clin Transplant. 2012;26(5):684-93.
74. Bucci JR, Matsumoto CS, Swanson SJ, et al. Donor hepatitis C seropositivity: clinical correlates and effect on early graft and patient survival in adult cadaveric kidney transplantation. J Am Soc Nephrol. 2004;15(12):2974-82.
75. Rao PS, Gallentine ML, Schaubel, et al. A comprehensive risk quantification score for deceased donor kidneys: the kidney donor risk index. Transplantation. 2009; 88(2):231-6.
76. Woodside KJ, Merion RM, Leichtman AB, et al. Utilization of kidneys with similar kidney donor risk index values from standard versus expanded criteria donors. Am J Transplant. 2012;12(8):2106-14.
77. A guide to calculating and interpreting the Kidney Donor Profile Index (KDPI). http://optn.transplant.hrsa.gov
78. Friedewald JJ. Utilization and outcomes of marginal kidneys – using Kidney Donor Risk Index to move beyond the current labels. Am J Transplant. 2012; 12(8):1971-2.

Advances in Minimally Invasive Techniques of Living Donor Nephrectomy

CHAPTER

2

Anthony C Watkins

ABSTRACT

It is well-established that the best outcomes in kidney transplant belong to those who undergo living renal donor transplant. Even the very first successful kidney transplant occurred because a living donor gave a kidney to his twin brother. Progress has been made over the past 60 years in the field of transplant to improve outcomes, but a severe organ shortage still remains. Living donation now accounts for nearly half of all renal transplants. However, it has only been since the 1990s that a significant rise in the number of living donors occurred. This coincides with the development of laparoscopic surgery and its application to transplant. The morbidity of open nephrectomy served as a disincentive that has largely been mitigated by minimally invasive techniques. This chapter examines the history of live donation and the progression of technologic innovation that has served to overcome barriers.

INTRODUCTION

The living donor nephrectomy has been instrumental to the success of kidney transplantation dating back to the first kidney transplant performed at the Peter Bent Brigham Hospital in 1954. During this historical procedure, an identical twin donated a kidney to his brother marking the inception of renal transplantation and specifically living donor transplantation. Despite the success of this landmark surgery outcomes were generally poor. Over the next several decades, advances in organ preservation and recovery, as well as tissue typing techniques helped lead to the proliferation of cadaveric donors. While cadaveric transplants played a vital role in increasing organ supply, over time the number of cadaveric kidneys available for transplantation has remained relatively stable, whereas the number of patients awaiting kidney transplantation has been expanding, thereby creating an increasing shortage of kidneys for patients.

Living donation represents the largest potential for increasing the donor pool and has many advantages over cadaveric donors including the elimination of prolonged waiting times and improved graft function representing the single best form of therapy for end-stage renal disease.[1,2] Initial rates of living donation were remarkably low at least in part due to the donor surgery. During an open-donor nephrectomy, the kidney is excised through an 8 to 9-in. flank incision along with removal of a rib.[3] Additional disincentives for potential donors included the length of hospitalization, postoperative pain, cosmetic concerns, and prolonged convalescence.[4] These concerns were mitigated when innovative surgical approaches using minimally invasive techniques altered the approach for the donor nephrectomy.

LAPAROSCOPIC DONOR NEPHRECTOMY

Minimally invasive techniques began to dramatically change the general surgical landscape by the 1980s by significantly reducing the length of incisions and introducing the concept of video-assisted techniques to perform surgery. After the laparoscopic removal of the gallbladder was replicated and became the gold standard for cholecystectomy, virtually every intra-abdominal organ quickly became targets to deploy this new technology including laparoscopic nephrectomy for renal tumors.[5] Living organ donors are the only surgical patients who derive no medical benefit from their procedure and hospitalization; therefore, the goal of the transplant team is to minimize short- and long-term effects from surgery. The concept of minimally invasive surgery had the potential to have a profound impact on these patients in these regards. A team at Johns Hopkins adopted this technique and reported the first human living laparoscopic donor nephrectomy (LDN) in 1995.[6] Although slight modifications were later made to the original procedure, LDN is commonly performed with the patient in the modified lateral decubitus position, with the side of kidney being procured in the elevated position (Fig. 2.1). Several small 5 to 15 mm ports are placed and the major steps include mobilizing the colon to expose the kidney and dissection of the ureter and kidney, including the hilum to maximize the length of the renal arteries and veins. Several different coagulation devices designed specifically for laparoscopy can be used for dissection and the renal arteries and veins are transected with the use of vascular staplers. The kidney is then removed through an additional incision measuring approximately 5 cm. The location for this incision can be placed in the epigastrium or more commonly as a Pfannenstiel incision. Early studies demonstrated that this laparoscopic technique is well-tolerated by patients with decreased morbidity, shorter hospital stay, and superior cosmetic results in comparison to the open approach.[4,7] Alternative approaches have been numerous with early reporting of successful retroperitoneal endoscopic and hand-assisted techniques.[8,9] The hand-assisted LDN, for example, utilizes an 8 cm midline incision and an occlusive sleeve to maintain pneumoperitoneum, while the laparoscopic procedure is performed. This sleeve allows the operation to be facilitated by manual assistance, which takes advantage throughout the procedure of the incision that is necessary for intact organ removal (Fig. 2.2).

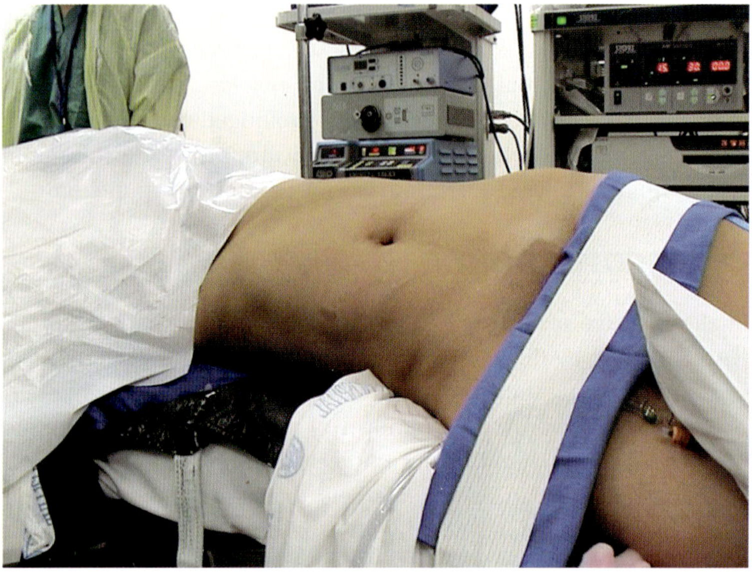

Fig. 2.1: Laparoscopic donor nephrectomy positioning. Patient is placed in the modified lateral decubitus position, with the side of kidney being procured in the elevated position.

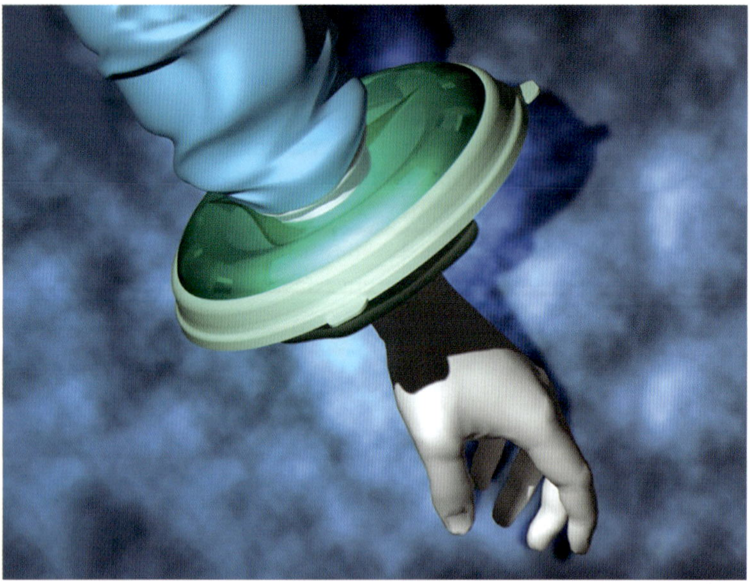

Fig. 2.2: Hand Port. An occlusive sleeve is used to maintain pneumoperitoneum while the laparoscopic procedure is being performed.

Despite variations in aspects such as port placement and the use of hand assistance, the concept of the minimally invasive approach with smaller incisions remains the cornerstone for these procedures.

Much like the impact minimally invasive techniques had on general surgery, the LDN marked the beginning of a new era for renal transplantation. Studies documenting equivalent complication rates and graft function compared to the open technique led to an increase in living donation.[3,10,11] In fact, by 2001 the number of live donor renal transplantations surpassed the deceased donor transplants for the first time and nearly doubled between 1996 and 2006.[12,13] While donor deaths have occurred worldwide, a recent series of >1000 LDNs without a donor death has been reported, further reinforcing the safety of this procedure for this subset of patients who have only emotional, and no medical, benefit to gain.[14] Unexpected benefits include an increase in nondirected donation by altruistic donors and paired kidney exchange.[15]

In spite of the tremendous response following the advent of LDN, there has been a recent decline in the total number of living kidney transplants coupled with an ever-growing waiting list.[13] The cause of this decline is likely multifactorial; however, fortunately efforts have been made to further modify LDN by utilizing even smaller incisions and developing other novel approaches to further decrease morbidity and hasten recovery. It is possible that these modifications will continue to make living donation more attractive to potential donors.

LAPAROENDOSCOPIC SINGLE-SITE SURGERY

Although conventional laparoscopy is less morbid than open surgery, it still requires several incisions, each at least 1–2 cm in length, and each incision carries potential morbidity risks of bleeding, pain, hernia, and/or internal organ damage with decreased cosmesis.[16,17] Laparoendoscopic single-site (LESS) surgery represents the next step in the evolution of standard laparoscopic surgery. LESS is employed using unique devices in which the laparoscopic camera and working instrument ports are contained allowing dissection and extraction through a single small entry into the abdomen. Laparoendoscopic single site donor nephrectomy (LESS-DN) uses this approach to dissect and remove the kidney through a single incision. At our institution, a single access GelPOINT device is inserted into the abdomen through a 4–5 cm periumbilical incision (Fig. 2.3). A bariatric laparoscope with a single light cord in parallel is used since traditional cords with perpendicular insertions into the scope greatly interfere with other instruments and surgeon movement (Fig. 2.4). Left LESS-DN is performed using three trocars through the device, while the right LESS-DN requires the placement of an additional port through the device for liver retraction. No extraumbilical ports are used.

The application of LESS-DN has been designed to improve on conventional LDN while maintaining equivalent outcomes. In addition to the

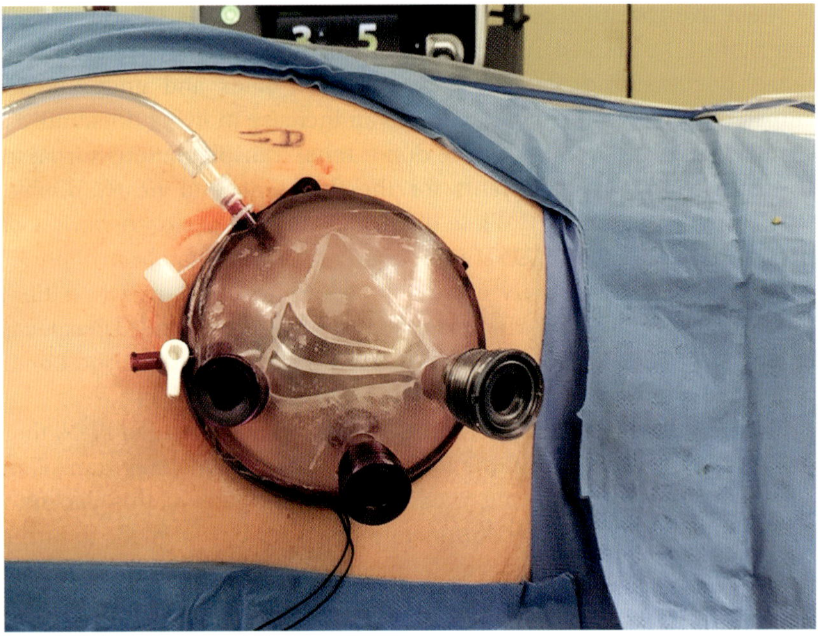

Fig. 2.3: GelPOINT™ Device. A single access GelPOINT™ device is inserted into the abdomen through a 4 to 5 cm periumbilical incision.

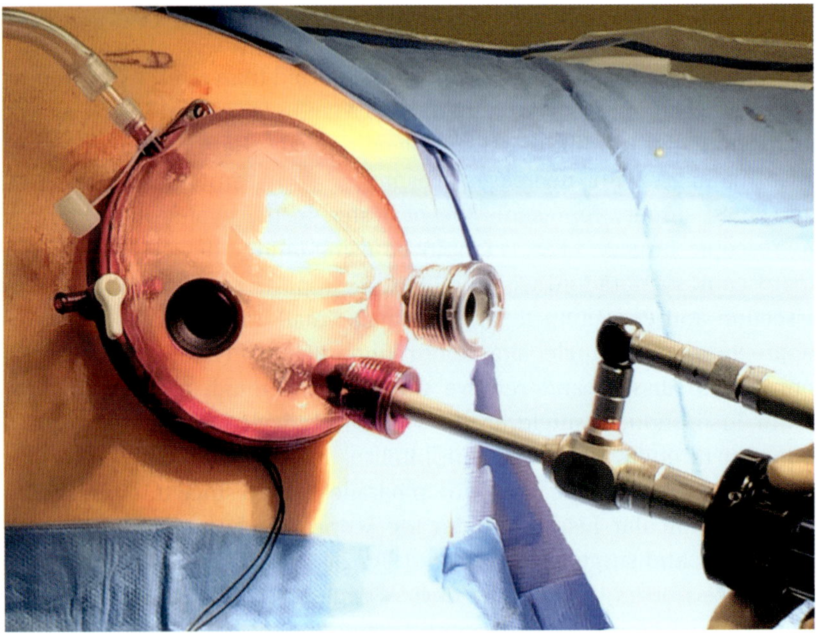

Fig. 2.4: Bariatric laparoscope. A bariatric laparoscope with a single light cord in parallel is used since traditional cords with perpendicular insertions into the scope greatly interfere with other instruments and surgeon movement.

potential benefits of cosmesis, other theoretical advantages of LESS-DN include less postoperative pain, faster recovery, and improvements in perioperative outcomes or other short-term measures of convalescence. While some studies comparing LESS-DN to conventional LDN have shown similar patient perioperative outcomes and an equivalent complication rates to LDN, other reports have suggested that there is less need for oral pain medication, fewer days off work, and fewer days to 100% physical recovery.[18-21] Ramasamy et al. found a shorter hospital stay, less estimated blood loss, and a marginally lower mean warm ischemia time in the LESS-DN group.[22] There were longer operative times in the LESS-DN group; however, more importantly, at 30 days there was no difference in the overall complication rate between the two groups. These findings suggest that with appropriate surgeon experience, LESS-DN can be safely done with equivalent if not superior outcomes. Longer operative times are partly due to the fact that LESS-DN is more technically challenging than standard laparoscopy secondary to decreased working space and lack of instrument triangulation, making dissection less ergonomic. This is particularly pronounced when harvesting allografts in patients with a BMI >30 kg/m^2 or with multiple renal arteries. Since patient safety is paramount, the placement of additional trocars is advisable when extreme difficulty in dissection is encountered. Articulating instruments have been used to aid in dissection and overcome the limitations of the smaller operative space; however, most are still in developmental stages.[23] It is possible that this approach will continue to become more prevalent as surgeon experience increases and improved instrumentation is developed.

ROBOTIC-ASSISTED DONOR NEPHRECTOMY

Although several advantages have been noted in comparison to open surgery, limitations of standard laparoscopy include two-dimensional imaging, restricted instrument motion, and limited surgeon comfort.[24,25] The da Vinci Surgical System (Intuitive Surgical, Inc., Sunnyvale, CA) combines robotics and computer imaging to enable microsurgery in a laparoscopic environment. The system consists of a surgeon's viewing and control console integrated with a high-performance, three-dimensional (3D) monitor system and a patient side cart consisting of three robotic arms: one arm allows positioning of the laparoscope with its two optic systems, whereas the other two arms allow placement of a variety of articulating instruments and behave as right and left surgeon hands (Figs. 2.5 and 2.6). The software within the da Vinci Surgical System translates the surgeon's hand, wrist, and finger movements into corresponding micromovements within the patient's body without any time delay.[26] This technology is felt to be a superior alternative

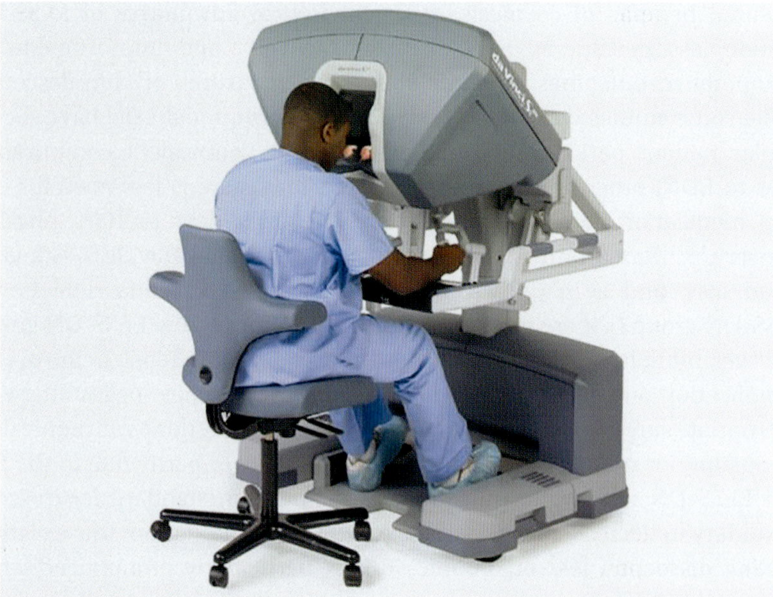

Fig. 2.5: da Vinci surgical system console. The da Vinci surgical system (Intuitive Surgical, Inc., Sunnyvale, CA) combines robotics and computer imaging to enable microsurgery in a laparoscopic environment. Pictured is the surgeon's viewing and control console.

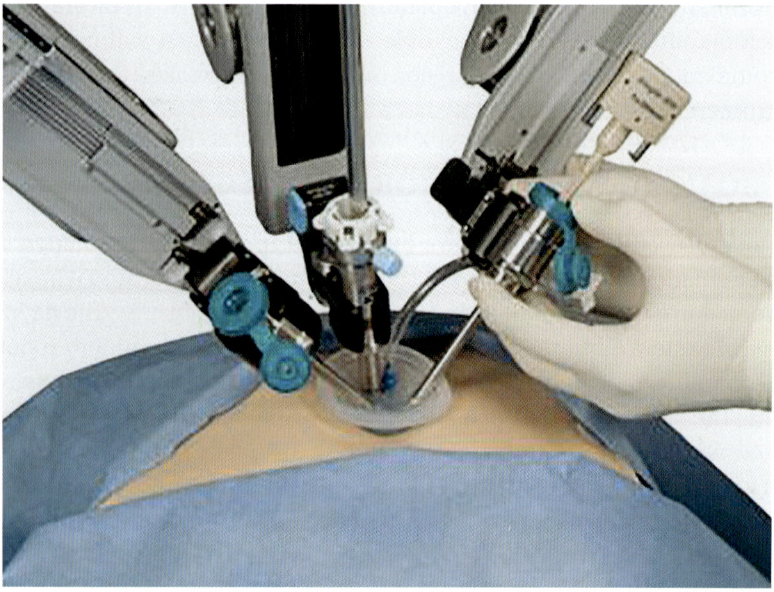

Fig. 2.6: da Vinci surgical system robotic arms. Pictured is patient side cart consisting of three robotic arms: one arm allows positioning of the laparoscope with its two optic systems, whereas the other two arms allow placement of a variety of articulating instruments and behave as right and left surgeon hands.

to traditional laparoscopy because of its ability to provide these endowrist instruments and 3D visualization of the operative field, thus maximizing the benefits and diminishing the possible risks and complications of living donor nephrectomy. Various reports have confirmed the feasibility of robotic-assisted nephrectomy for living-donor kidney transplantation, even in the presence of multiple renal arteries.[24,25,27–29] The robotic hand-assisted donor nephrectomy (RHADN), e.g., has been used extensively by the team at University of Illinois at Chicago where they have found it be a safe and effective procedure.[26,27,30] Similar to the hand-assisted LDN approach, the patient is placed in the right decubitus position and a hand port is placed in a 7 cm infraumbilical incision for manual assistance and future kidney retrieval. Four 8–12 mm trocars are then placed for the robotic-assisted portion of the procedure. In their experience, RHADN is faster when compared with standard LDN without associated increased risks to the patient.[27]

Other groups have integrated previous experience gained with LESS, natural orifice transluminal surgery (NOTES), and robotics to perform various hybrid procedures.[31,32] NOTES is a relatively recent concept that refers to surgery performed through natural orifices (vagina, mouth, rectum) for the purpose of eliminating external scars and minimizing pain.[33] Part of this reduction in pain is theoretically derived from a different pattern of innervation of internal organs compared to incisions through the abdominal wall. Kaouk et al. described a novel surgical approach by performing a transvaginal hybrid NOTES robotic donor nephrectomy.[31] With this procedure a Single Incision Laparoscopic Surgery (SILS) port and an 8 mm trocar were placed through the same umbilical incision, while a GelPOINT port was placed transvaginally via the posterior fornix. The authors report that the clashing and difficult working angles experienced during the standard LESS-DN approach were overcome by placing the second robotic arm through this vaginal port. The kidney was removed via an endoscopic retrieval bag inserted through the GelPOINT. No complications occurred and the donor was discharged after 48 hours without incident and similarly good recipient outcome noted.[31] Challenges with the robot approach include its learning curve and further experience needed to compare cost and outcomes to standard LDN to determine that procedure is safer and more cost-effective. Superiority of one minimally invasive technique over another is unlikely to ever be proven, as outcomes likely relate predominantly to the individual surgeon comfort and experience.

DONOR EVALUATION AND SURGICAL CONSIDERATIONS

The donor evaluation involves a complete medical, surgical, and psychosocial workup to ensure both donor safety and recipient benefit. The donor surgeon's goal during the evaluation process is to minimize any potential morbidity and mortality associated with the operation paying particular attention to the anatomy and function of the donor kidneys.

Preoperative imaging is an essential part of the donor evaluation and typically involves computed tomography (CT) angiography with vascular reconstruction to allow adequate assessment of arterial, venous, and renal parenchymal anatomy in addition to the surrounding organs.[34] Magnetic resonance angiography can also be used as an alternative. The left kidney is typically procured because the longer left renal vein makes the operation for both the donor and recipient easier; however, the goal of the transplant team is to leave the donor with the best kidney, therefore other factors have to be examined.[35] For example, if a size discrepancy of ≥1 cm exists between the kidneys, additional functional studies should be performed including renal scintigraphy or calculations based on 3D CT reconstructions to rule out any functional differences between the kidneys.[36] The vascular anatomy must also be evaluated because identification of multiple arteries, small polar arteries and anomalous venous anatomy may influence the choice of kidney.

Although no absolute contraindications exists in regards to a maximum BMI have not been defined, many centers have respective cutoffs since obesity can lead to a more technically challenging procedure due to an increased amount of intra-abdominal fat and is a surrogate for poor health.[37] In addition, adhesions from previous abdominal surgery can add a significant level of difficulty to the donor operation and old incisions should be assessed to determine if planned approach should be modified accordingly. For example, previous pelvic surgery may influence the location of the incision used for kidney retrieval (i.e. epigastrium vs Pfannenstiel). In our experience, there has been a low rate of converting from LESS-DN to an open procedure.[38] Minimally invasive donor surgery can be applied as long as the health of the donor remains the primary focus.

CONCLUSION

While the surgical aspect of the recipient renal transplant has not evolved dramatically, there has been much progress made in the evolution of the living donor nephrectomy. With the advent of minimally invasive techniques, the transplant community has been able to minimize the morbidity associated with living donation by providing faster recovery, decreasing hospital stays and improving cosmesis while maintaining excellent graft outcomes. As we continue to face a significant discrepancy between organ supply and demand, further advances in these techniques have the potential to foster a greater increase in live donations.

REFERENCES

1. Jofre R, Lopez-Gomez JM, Moreno F, et al. Changes in quality of life after renal transplantation. Am J Kidney Dis. 1998;32(1):93-100.
2. Laupacis A, Keown P, Pus N, et al. A study of the quality of life and cost-utility of renal transplantation. Kidney Int. 1996;50(1):235-42.
3. Ruiz-Deya G, Cheng S, Palmer E, et al. Open donor, laparoscopic donor and hand assisted laparoscopic donor nephrectomy: a comparison of outcomes. J Urol. 2001;166(4):1270-3. Discussion 1273-4.
4. Ratner LE, Kavoussi LR, Schulam PG, et al. Comparison of laparoscopic live donor nephrectomy versus the standard open approach. Transplant Proc. 1997;29(1-2):138-9.
5. Clayman RV, Kavoussi LR, Soper NJ, et al. Laparoscopic nephrectomy. N Engl J Med. 19919;324(19):1370-1.
6. Ratner LE, Ciseck LJ, Moore RG, et al. Laparoscopic live donor nephrectomy. Transplant J. 1995;60(9):1047-9.
7. Flowers JL, Jacobs S, Cho E, et al. Comparison of open and laparoscopic live donor nephrectomy. Ann Surg. 1997;226(4):483-9. Discussion 489-90.
8. Yang SC, Park DS, Lee DH, et al. Retroperitoneal endoscopic live donor nephrectomy: Report of 3 cases. J Urol. 1995;153(6):1884-6.
9. Wolf JS, Tchetgen MB, Merion RM. Hand-assisted laparoscopic live donor nephrectomy. Urology. 1998;52(5):885-7.
10. Matas AJ, Bartlett ST, Leichtman AB, et al. Morbidity and mortality after living kidney donation, 1999-2001: survey of United States transplant centers. Am J Transplant. 2003;3(7):830-4.
11. Eng M. The role of laparoscopic donor nephrectomy in renal transplantation. Am Surg. 2010;76(4):349-53.
12. Schweitzer EJ, Wilson J, Jacobs S, et al. Increased rates of donation with laparoscopic donor nephrectomy. Ann Surg. 2000;232(3):392-400.
13. SRTR, OPTN. Kidney chapter, 2010 SRTR & OPTN Annual Data Report. 2012; 24:1-36.
14. Ahearn AJ, Posselt AM, Kang S-M, et al. Experience with laparoscopic donor nephrectomy among more than 1000 cases low complication rates, despite more challenging cases: archives of surgery. Am Med Assoc. 2011;146(7):859-64.
15. Leeser DB, Aull MJ, Afaneh C, et al. Living donor kidney paired donation transplantation: experience as a founding member center of the National Kidney Registry. Clin Transplant. 2012;26(3):E213-22.
16. Lowry PS, Moon TD, D'Alessandro A, et al. Symptomatic port-site hernia associated with a non-bladed trocar after laparoscopic live-donor nephrectomy. J Endourol. 2003;17(7):493-4.
17. Marcovici I. Significant abdominal wall hematoma from an umbilical port insertion. JSLS. 2001;5(3):293-5.
18. Raman JD, Bagrodia A, Cadeddu JA. Single-Incision, umbilical laparoscopic versus conventional laparoscopic nephrectomy: a comparison of perioperative outcomes and short-term measures of convalescence. Eur Urol. 2009;55(5):1198-1206.
19. Andonian S, Rais-Bahrami S, Atalla MA, et al. Laparoendoscopic single-site Pfannenstiel versus standard laparoscopic donor nephrectomy. J Endourol. 2010;24(3):429-32.
20. Canes D, Berger A, Aron M, et al. Laparo-endoscopic single site (LESS) versus standard laparoscopic left donor nephrectomy: matched-pair comparison. Eur Urol. 2010;57(1):95-101.

21. Afaneh C, Aull MJ, Gimenez E, et al. Comparison of laparoendoscopic single-site donor nephrectomy and conventional laparoscopic donor nephrectomy: donor and recipient outcomes. Urology. 2011;78(6):1332-7.
22. Ramasamy R, Afaneh C, Katz M, et al. Comparison of complications of laparoscopic versus laparoendoscopic single site donor nephrectomy using the modified Clavien grading system. J Urol. 2011;186(4):1386-90.
23. Raman JD, Bensalah K, Bagrodia A, et al. Laboratory and clinical development of single keyhole umbilical nephrectomy. Urology. 2007;70(6):1039-42.
24. Hubert J, Renoult E, Mourey E, et al. Complete robotic-assistance during laparoscopic living donor nephrectomies: an evaluation of 38 procedures at a single site. Int J Urol. 2007;14(11):986-9.
25. Pietrabissa A, Abelli M, Spinillo A, et al. Robotic-assisted laparoscopic donor nephrectomy with transvaginal extraction of the kidney. Am J Transplant. 2010;10(12):2708-11.
26. Horgan S, Vanuno D, Sileri P, et al. Robotic-assisted laparoscopic donor nephrectomy for kidney transplantation. Transplant J. 2002;73(9):1474-9.
27. Horgan S, Galvani C, Gorodner MV, et al. Effect of robotic assistance on the 'learning curve' for laparoscopic hand-assisted donor nephrectomy. Surg Endosc. 2007;21(9):1512-17.
28. Gorodner V, Horgan S, Galvani C, et al. Routine left robotic-assisted laparoscopic donor nephrectomy is safe and effective regardless of the presence of vascular anomalies. Transplant Int. 2006;19(8):636-40.
29. Giacomoni A, Di Sandro S, Lauterio A, et al. Initial experience with robot-assisted nephrectomy for living-donor kidney transplantation: feasibility and technical notes. Transplant Proc. 2013;45(7):2627-31.
30. Horgan S, Benedetti E, Moser F. Robotically assisted donor nephrectomy for kidney transplantation. Am J Surg. 2004;188(4A Suppl):45S–51S.
31. Kaouk JH, Khalifeh A, Laydner H, et al. Transvaginal hybrid natural orifice transluminal surgery robotic donor nephrectomy: first clinical application. Urology. 2012;80(6):1171-5.
32. Allaf ME, Singer A, Shen W, et al. Laparoscopic live donor nephrectomy with vaginal extraction: initial report. Am J Transplant. 2010;10(6):1473-7.
33. Marescaux J, Dallemagne B, Perretta S, et al. Surgery without scars: report of transluminal cholecystectomy in a human being. Arch Surg. 2007;142(9):823-6. Discussion 826-7.
34. Pozniak MA, Balison DJ, Lee FTJ, et al. CT angiography of potential renal transplant donors. Radiographics. 1998;18(3):565-87.
35. Ratner LE, Kavoussi LR, Chavin KD, et al. Laparoscopic live donor nephrectomy: technical considerations and allograft vascular length. Transplant J. 1998;65(12): 1657-8.
36. Summerlin AL, Lockhart ME, Strang AM, et al. Determination of split renal function by 3D reconstruction of CT angiograms: a comparison with gamma camera renography. AJR Am J Roentgenol. 2008;191(5):1552-8.
37. Kok NFM, IJzermans JNM, Schouten O, et al. Laparoscopic donor nephrectomy in obese donors: easier to implement in overweight women? Transpl Int. 2007;20(11):956-61.
38. Wang GJ, Afaneh C, Aull M, et al. Laparoendoscopic single site live donor nephrectomy: single institution report of initial 100 cases. J Urol. 2011;186(6):2333-7.

Kidney Paired Donation as a Strategy to Increase Living Donor Kidney Transplantation

CHAPTER 3

Meredith J Aull, Sandip Kapur

ABSTRACT

Kidney paired donation (KPD) is a mechanism designed to provide kidney transplant candidates with willing but incompatible living donors the ability to enroll in a registry of other incompatible pairs in order to find a compatible transplant. Blood-type incompatible, crossmatch incompatible, and compatible donor-recipient pairs may benefit from transplantation facilitated by KPD. For highly sensitized kidney transplant candidates, desensitization therapy in combination with KPD offers an important option. KPD represents the most promising resource available to increase the number of kidneys available for transplantation due to the ongoing shortage of deceased donor organs.

INTRODUCTION

It was estimated that about 2 million people worldwide would have end-stage renal disease by 2010.[1] On January 17, 2014, >99,000 patients in the United States were on the United Network for Organ Sharing (UNOS) waiting list for a kidney transplant from a deceased donor.[2] It is presumed that the vast majority of these patients have no potential living donors, or have willing but incompatible donors and are unaware of the KPD option. Prior to the introduction of KPD, blood type (ABO) and/or immunologic incompatibility has limited living donor kidney transplantation.

Based on overall blood-type distributions in the United States, approximately one of every three potential living kidney donors is blood-type incompatible with their intended recipient. Immunologic incompatibility, as evidenced by a positive crossmatch and development of donor-specific antibody (DSA), occurs when transplant candidates are exposed to non-self (foreign) human leukocyte antigens (HLA) through blood transfusion, pregnancy, and/or prior transplantation. Exposure to foreign HLA leads many patients to develop anti-HLA antibodies, leading to reactivity against potential organ donors (DSA). Patients with a high degree of sensitization (i.e. a high antibody load/high DSA levels) often cannot find an organ donor against whom they do not have a significant immunologic reaction, which might lead to early and severe rejection of the allograft if transplantation were to occur. In the United States, approximately 40% of adult patients awaiting a kidney transplant have some degree of sensitization against HLA, while about 10% are considered highly sensitized, defined as a panel reactive antibody level above 80%.[3]

Although successful transplantation using ABO incompatible donors or by transplanting across a positive crossmatch is possible,[4,5] these methods do not necessarily represent the best solution for patients with incompatible donors. Both incompatible transplantation methods require "desensitization," which requires the use of interventions such as plasmapheresis, intravenous immunoglobulin (IVIG), rituximab, splenectomy and/or mycophenolate mofetil to reduce anti-ABO (anti-A or anti-B) or anti-HLA titers in order to enable transplantation between the incompatible donor and recipient. The excess immunosuppression, morbidity [via increased risk of antibody-mediated rejection (ABMR) and its associated treatment], and cost associated with incompatible transplants leave room for alternative solutions.[6,7] A meeting report from a Roche Organ Transplantation Research Foundation-organized symposium agreed that the goal of the transplant community should be to prevent ABMR rather than treat it once it occurs in order to avoid the negative consequences of ABMR on the transplant allograft.[7]

KIDNEY PAIRED DONATION: A SOLUTION TO THE SHORTAGE OF ORGANS FOR TRANSPLANT

The concept of paired exchange, as a mechanism to facilitate living donor kidney transplantation, was first introduced by Rapaport in 1996 as a potential solution to the shortage of deceased donor organs.[8] Rapaport proposed an international registry where eligible and willing, but blood-type incompatible donors could donate via organ exchange facilitated through this registry. Donors would undergo simultaneous nephrectomy, donated organs would be transported via courier, and transplantation into the recipients would occur simultaneously.

Almost two decades after the concept was first introduced, paired exchange had become a somewhat routine occurrence at a few transplant centers.[9,10] The logistical issues associated with international exchanges, such as those proposed by Rapaport, have not yet been fully solved; however, an international exchange has been reported between the Unites States and Canada.[11] National exchange programs have been successfully developed in Korea,[9] the Netherlands,[10] and the United States.[12,13] Most importantly, the concept has dramatically evolved from simple exchanges between two incompatible donor-recipient pairs to complex chains consisting of up to 30 incompatible pairs.[14] A 2012 consensus conference described KPD as an "elegant but complex solution" to the shortage of organs available

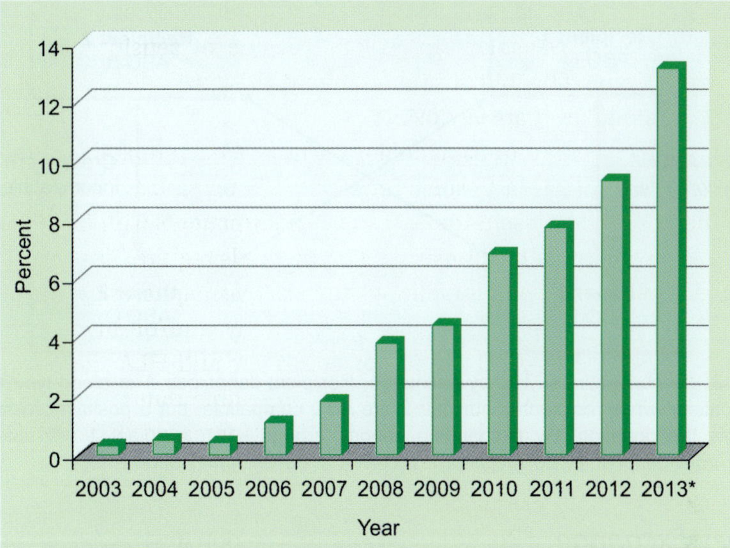

Fig. 3.1: Percent of living donor transplants from paired donation in the United States. *2013 data includes transplants performed through 31/10/2013.

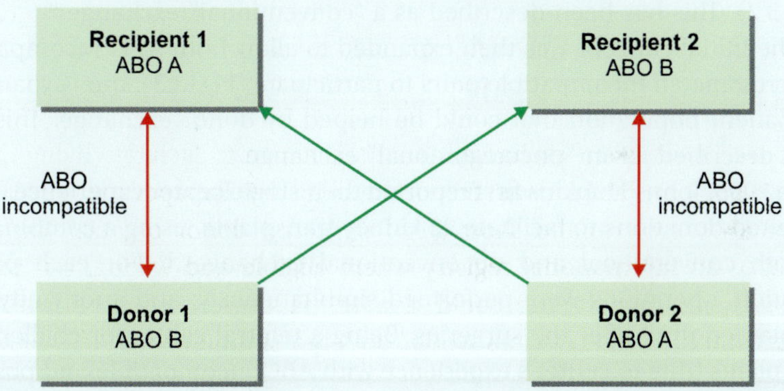

Fig. 3.2: "Conventional" kidney exchange. Recipient-donor pair 1 and recipient-donor pair 2 are both blood-type (ABO) incompatible. By exchanging donors through KPD, recipient 1 will receive a kidney from donor 2, while recipient 2 receives a kidney from donor 1.

for transplant.[15] As seen in Figure 3.1, paired donation has facilitated an increasing percentage of living donor kidney transplants in the United States over the past decade.[2]

Kidney Paired Donation Models

The initial concept proposed by Rapaport has rapidly progressed into much more complex exchanges. The types of exchanges are described in this chapter, and are illustrated, from simple to complex, in Figures 3.2 through 3.6.

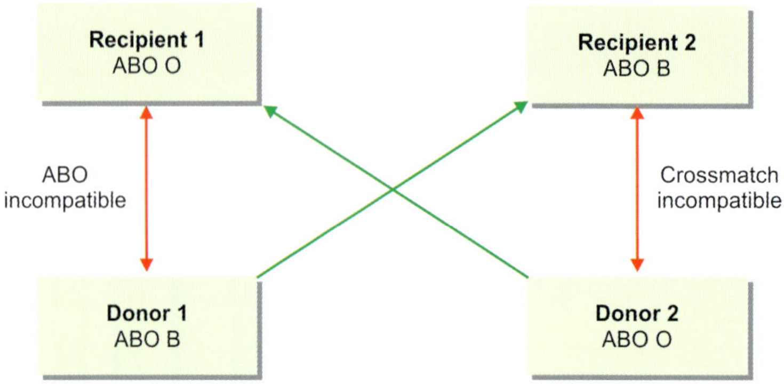

Fig. 3.3: "Unconventional" kidney exchange. Recipient-donor pair 1 is blood-type (ABO) incompatible, while recipient-donor pair 2 are ABO compatible, but a positive crossmatch prevents the donation. By exchanging donors through KPD, recipient 1 will receive a kidney from donor 2, while recipient 2 receives a kidney from donor 1.

Kidney Exchange

As first described by Rapaport, kidney exchange occurred between two blood-type incompatible donor-recipient pairs, who through participation in an exchange, were matched to create ABO compatible transplants (Fig. 3.2). This has been described as a "conventional" exchange.[16]

The initial concept was then expanded to allow both ABO incompatible and crossmatch incompatible pairs to participate (Fig. 3.3), thus expanding the patient population that could be helped by donor exchange. This has been described as an "unconventional" exchange.[16]

In 2005, Johns Hopkins first reported their single center experience using 10 paired donations to facilitate 22 kidney transplants, using a combination of both conventional and unconventional exchanges.[16] For each paired donation, operations were performed simultaneously, and anonymity was maintained until after the surgeries. Being a referral center for challenging transplants (due to center's experience with ABO incompatible and positive crossmatch transplants), the Hopkins experience is particularly notable for its success in transplanting within their difficult-to-match pool of transplant candidates.

List Exchange

List exchange (Fig. 3.4) allows the incompatible donor of a donor-recipient pair to donate their kidney to the deceased donor waiting list, and in exchange, their intended recipient receives priority on the deceased donor waiting list. Critics of this model point out that the majority of pairs participating in such an exchange will be blood-type incompatible, with an ABO non-O donor and an ABO O recipient, which is unfair to the ABO O recipients on the waiting list who will have to wait longer for an ABO O deceased donor kidney.

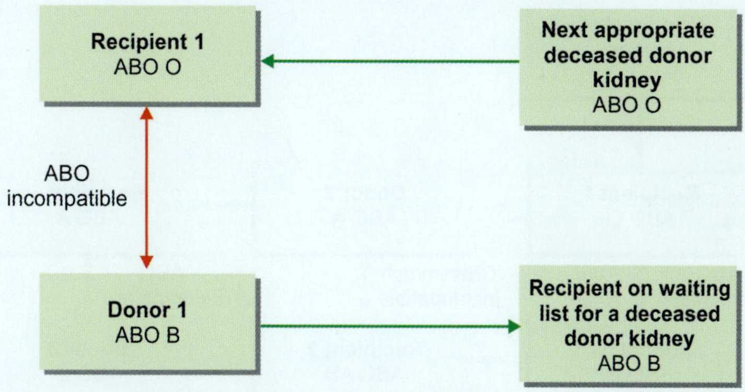

Fig. 3.4: List exchange. Recipient-donor pair 1 are blood-type (ABO) incompatible. In list exchange, the incompatible living donor donates a kidney to a patient on the waiting list for a deceased donor kidney. Then, the original intended recipient receives priority for the next appropriate deceased donor kidney.

In 2004, representatives from transplant centers in the United States UNOS Region 1 (New England) reported on implementation of a living donor/list exchange program, which had facilitated 17 transplants by the end of 2003.[17]

Domino Paired Donation

The domino paired donation (DPD) model (also called a "closed" chain) begins with donation by a nondirected donor (NDD), also known as an altruistic or "Good Samaritan" donor (Fig. 3.5). NDDs are living kidney donors who choose to donate despite not having an intended recipient for their kidney. The first reported kidney donation by a NDD occurred in the United States in August 1999.[18] By representing the general population, these NDDs present an important source of blood type O donors. This initial donation starts a "chain" of transplants where the NDD kidney recipient's intended but incompatible donor is matched to a compatible recipient, then that recipient's intended but incompatible donor is matched with a compatible recipient, and so on. If a compatible recipient cannot be found for the last donor's kidney within the KPD registry, the kidney is allocated to the deceased donor waiting list according to UNOS policy, and the chain ends (thus the term "closed" chain).

After successfully implementing KPD in the mid-1990s, the Korean KPD program began utilizing DPD in 2001, and performed 179 transplants as a result between 2001 and 2007.[19] Seventy transplant chains, the majority of which transplanted 2 or 3 patients, were initiated by an altruistic donor, and the last kidney went to a patient without a living donor. Donors traveled to the recipient transplant center, and operations were not simultaneous, but did occur within a short time frame (goal <7 days). In the United States,

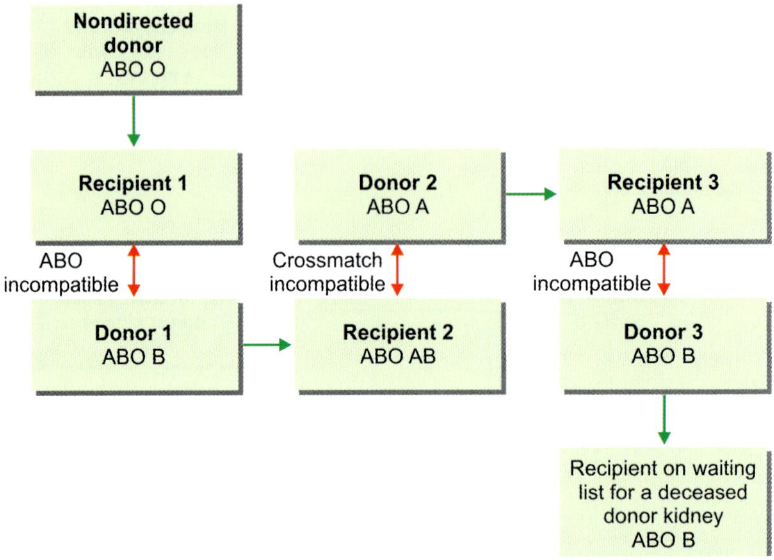

Fig. 3.5: Domino paired donation. Recipient-donor pairs 1 and 3 are blood-type (ABO) incompatible, while recipient-donor pair 2 is crossmatch incompatible. In Domino paired donation, a nondirected (altruistic) donor begins a chain of transplants by donating to recipient 1; recipient 1's donor (1) then donates to recipient 2, recipient 2's donor (2) donates to recipient 3, and recipient 3's donor (3) donates a kidney to a patient on the waiting list for a deceased donor kidney; the chain then ends.

Montgomery and colleagues first proposed the use of NDDs to generate multiple transplants via DPD in 2006.[20] Roth and colleagues performed simulations that showed that utilizing NDDs to start chains of transplants in the DPD model could increase the number of kidneys available for transplant.[21]

Nonsimultaneous Extended Altruistic Donation

Similar to the DPD model, a transplant chain in the nonsimultaneous extended altruistic donation (NEAD) model (also referred to as an "open" chain) also begins with donation by a NDD (Fig. 3.6). Like the DPD model, the NDDs donation starts a chain of transplants where the NDD kidney recipient's intended but incompatible donor is matched to a compatible recipient, then that recipient's intended but incompatible donor is matched with a compatible recipient, and so on. If a compatible recipient (with a willing but incompatible living donor as opposed to a patient on the waiting list who has no potential donor) cannot be found for the last donor's kidney, the donor serves as a "bridge" donor who waits until a suitable recipient-donor pair enters the registry, and the chain continues on at a later date (thus the term "open" chain).

Rees and colleagues were the first to report use of a NEAD chain in 2009; the chain facilitated 10 living donor kidney transplants.[12] Their group

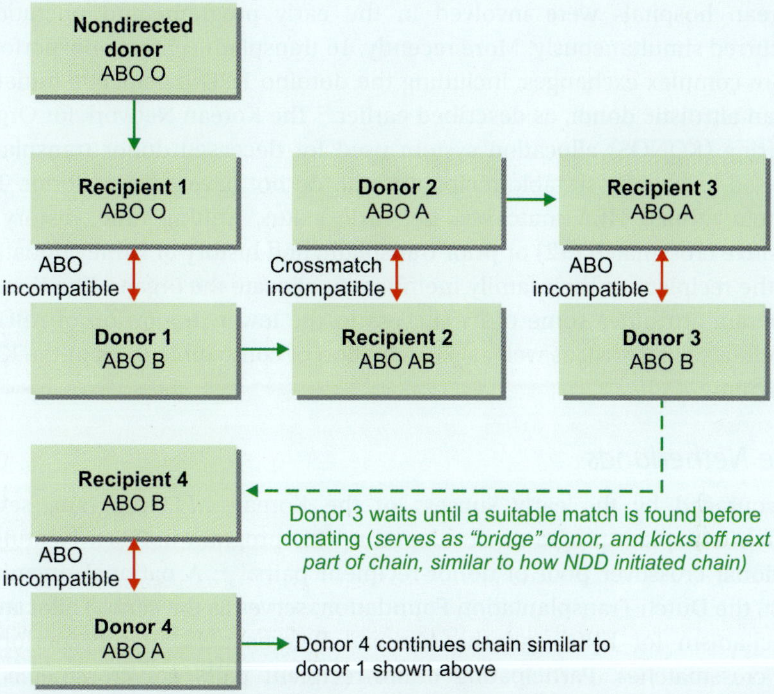

Fig. 3.6: NEAD (non-simultaneous extended altruistic donation). Recipient-donor pairs 1 and 3 are blood-type (ABO) incompatible, while recipient-donor pair 2 is crossmatch incompatible. In Domino paired donation, a nondirected (altruistic) donor begins a chain of transplants by donating to recipient 1; recipient 1's donor (1) then donates to recipient 2, recipient 2's donor (2) donates to recipient 3, and recipient 3's donor (3) then waits to donate until a suitable match is found within the KPD registry, and the chain continues at that time. Donor 3 is considered a "bridge" donor, and the donor's role in kicking off the continuation of the chain mimics that of the initial NDD.

combined several different techniques, including KPD combined with ABO incompatible transplantation and combined with desensitization, as well as participation of a compatible donor-recipient pair.

The National Kidney Registry (NKR) has had great success in transplanting patients via NEAD chains.[13] The NKR model represents a combination of NEAD and DPD; bridge donor characteristics guide the decision for that bridge donor to wait and start another transplant chain (e.g. if ABO O) vs donating to the waiting list (e.g. ABO AB or unable to wait to donate).

Active KPD Programs

Korea

The Korean KPD program was initiated for crossmatch incompatible pairs in 1991, and after early success, was expanded to include ABO incompatible pairs, as well as spousal pairs seeking a better genetic (HLA) match.[9] Three

Korean hospitals were involved in the early program, and operations occurred simultaneously. More recently, 16 transplant centers now perform more complex exchanges, including the domino KPD transplants initiated by an altruistic donor, as described earlier.[19] The Korean Network for Organ Sharing (KONOS) allocation system used for deceased donor transplants is used to identify suitable recipients who do not have a living donor. The system utilizes HLA matching, pediatric status, waiting time, history of positive crossmatch (>2) or prior transplant, and history of kidney donation by the recipient or their family members to allocate the organs. The Korean program attributes some of its success to the lower proportion of ABO O candidates in Korea, as well as participation of compatible pairs in the KPD program.

The Netherlands

Encouraged by the early success of the Korean KPD program, seven Dutch transplant programs developed a KPD program in 2004, creating a national crossover pool of donor-recipient pairs.[22,23] A national organization, the Dutch Transplantation Foundation, serves as the central allocation mechanism for KPD, and the National Reference Laboratory performs all crossmatches. Participating donor-recipient pairs are crossmatch or ABO incompatible, and the algorithm calculates the "match probability" or "MP" for each recipient, based on their degree of sensitization, blood type, and unacceptable HLA antigens (those against which the recipient has antibodies). Blood-type identical pairs are allocated first, in attempts to reserve ABO O donors for ABO O recipients, and the MP is then used to rank the recipients. More recently, de Klerk and colleagues describe the barriers faced by the Netherlands exchange program, which transplanted 46.3% of participants (128/276) between January 2004 and July 2008; all participants had incompatibility with their original intended donor.[10]

North America

There are several single and multicenter KPD Registries that are actively facilitating transplants today in North America, as described below. Although KPD has undergone significant growth in the United States within the past 6 years, a recent study showed that a limited number of transplant centers are responsible for the majority of transplants being facilitated by KPD.[24] This analysis showed that at the 10% of transplant centers with the highest rates of KPD, between 9.9% and 38.5% of those center's living donor kidney transplant volumes came from KPD participation between 2009 and 2011. Importantly, the study found that if all transplant centers participated in KPD in a similar fashion to these successful centers, >1,000 additional living donor kidney transplants could be generated each year in the United States.

Table 3.1: United States multicenter kidney paired donation programs

KPD program	*Transplants facilitated**	*Website*
Alliance for Paired Donation	22 (between 7/18/07 and unk/2010)[25]	http://www.paireddonation.org
Johns Hopkins	45 (between 2001 and 8/27/07)[26]	http://www.hopkinsmedicine.org/transplant/programs/kidney/incompatible/paired_kidney_exchange.html
National Kidney Registry	942 (between 2/14/2008 and 1/26/2014)[27]	http://www.kidneyregistry.org
North American Paired Donation Network	Not available	http://www.paireddonationnetwork.org
North Central Donor Exchange Cooperative	Not available	http://www.ncdec.org
United Network for Organ Sharing	68 (between 10/2010 and 11/4/2013)[28]	http://optn.transplant.hrsa.gov/resources/KPDPP.asp
Washington Regional Transplant Community	Not available	http://www.beadonor.org

*Transplants facilitated derived from published literature or publicly available sources.

Multicenter KPD in the United States

There are currently seven multicenter KPD programs functioning in the United States,[15] providing a driving force for competition and innovation among programs (Table 3.1). Despite the individual successes of these multicenter KPD programs, a single national KPD program is a proposed ultimate goal, as it would generate the largest pool of donor-recipient pairs and thus could facilitate more transplants. As compared to geographically smaller countries with a small number of transplant centers (such as the Netherlands and Korea), implementation of a national KPD program in the United States is understandably more challenging due to its size and >225 kidney transplant programs.[2]

As can be seen in Table 3.1, the NKR is the most successful KPD program in the United States, likely attributable to several factors. The NKR was founded by a father familiar with the struggles of finding a compatible living donor for his daughter, and who approached the problem from a new and different perspective. In addition, collaboration among many of the major United States' national kidney transplant programs (>65 centers as of January 2014[27]), utilization of advanced software to match donors with recipients, and transparent policies and procedures followed by all participating transplant centers (publicly available at www.kidneyregistry.org) have contributed to the success of NKR.

Single Center KPD in the United States

The kidney transplant program at Methodist San Antonio has been the most successful single center KPD program in the United States, having performed 134 kidney transplants over approximately 3 years.[29] This program includes incompatible donor-recipient pairs as well as compatible pairs with an age discrepancy and utilizes the database developed at Johns Hopkins for the purpose of matching donors and recipients for KPD. This program attributes its success (in spite of being a single center with a limited pool of donors and recipients) to prospective education of donor-recipient pairs about KPD, comprehensive immunological profiling of donor and recipient, flexible assignment of unacceptable antigens, storage of blood samples for future testing, use of desensitization, subtyping of ABO A donors, and inclusion of compatible pairs.

Multicenter KPD in Canada

In Canada, the Living Donor Paired Exchange kidney transplant registry is a partnership between Canadian Blood Services and transplant programs across the country designed to facilitate living kidney donations between patients with a willing but incompatible donor and other pairs in the same situation. The program, initially launched as a pilot program in 3 Canadian provinces in 2009, had performed 171 kidney transplants by October 2012.[30]

Other Countries

In addition to the programs mentioned above, there are also KPD programs in Australia,[31] the United Kingdom,[32] and Spain.[33]

CLINICAL OUTCOMES

Experience with KPD to date shows that transplants facilitated by KPD have equivalent outcomes compared to traditional living donor kidney transplantation.[13,16,23,26,34] These excellent outcomes are particularly impressive considering the extent of sensitization exhibited by many recipients in the registry pool. Patient and graft survival rates have been similar to those expected with traditional living unrelated kidney transplantation.

WHAT FACTORS HAVE DRIVEN THE INCREASE IN PAIRED DONATION FACILITATED TRANSPLANTS?

Keys to Success

Participation of Nondirected Donors

It is through the participation of NDDs that KPD programs have had greater success in facilitating transplants in recent years. By introducing a donor to the KPD pool who has no linked recipient, the pool of donors increases and mimics the characteristics of the general population, bringing much-needed ABO O donors into the pool. A recent analysis shows that utilization of NDDs for transplant chains has the ability to significantly amplify the benefit provided by NDDs, since each NDD generates an average of five transplants, or even more if the donor is ABO O.[35] Most KPD programs require psychiatric evaluation as part of the evaluation process for potential NDDs.

Large Pool Size

By having a large pool of incompatible donor-recipient pairs, there is an increased chance of finding an acceptable match. A large pool generally also increases the heterogenicity of the pool, which is beneficial in matching donors with recipients. In conjunction with the advanced software utilized by successful KPD programs, a larger pool can generate many more potential matches for incompatible pairs.[36]

Mathematical Modeling Software/Matching Algorithm

Many mathematical models have been developed to identify matches for the donor-recipient pairs participating in KPD registries. These models vary greatly in terms of the factors used in the model; however, most use similar criteria for determining matches. The frequency at which "match runs" occur also varies greatly among KPD programs.

The common factors include the following:

- Donor and recipient ABO type
- Virtual crossmatch results using donor HLA antigen and recipient anti-HLA antibody profile
- Preferences related to donor travel (i.e. distance willing to travel)
- Waiting time within KPD registry
- Limiting ABO O donors from donating to ABO non-O recipients
- Entering ABO A2 donors as ABO O* donors[37]

As more advanced software has been developed to facilitate KPD, there has been movement away from the traditional integer programming algorithms used in early models. For example, the NKR software is built upon technology utilizing concepts from capital market exchange systems.[36] In order to improve both the quantity and quality of transplants, an outcome-based strategy for generating matches within KPD has also been proposed.[38]

Much research has focused on the ability of the two newest KPD models (DPD vs NEAD) to generate the highest numbers of transplants. However, there does not yet appear to be a definitive answer due to the numerous factors involved in the modeling process.[39,40]

Virtual Crossmatch

The availability of advanced tools from the field of immunology has also been instrumental to the growth of KPD. Traditionally, a crossmatch is performed utilizing serum from both the potential organ donor and transplant candidate, and uses the complement-dependent cytotoxicity test and flow cytometry to detect antibodies that react with donor HLA antigens. An advanced method, called a virtual crossmatch, utilizes identified DSA titers/unacceptable antigens for a particular candidate (via screening with single antigen beads such as Luminex) and the detailed HLA typing of the potential donor to assess for potential reactivity. Virtual crossmatching has been successfully employed by several large KPD registries,[41,42] reducing logistical issues and cost associated with performing a traditional crossmatch. Traditional crossmatch testing is then performed between matched donor-recipient pairs in order to ensure compatibility prior to the scheduled transplant.

Flexible assignment of unacceptable antigens may be important,[29,43] particularly when attempting to identify potential donors for highly sensitized transplant candidates. By not excluding antigens to which the candidate has a low level of antibody, a KPD registry can increase the pool of potential donors for that recipient; this is where willingness to employ a combination of KPD and desensitization can increase success in identifying a suitable donor for a sensitized patient.

Willingness to Combine KPD with Desensitization Protocols

Montgomery and colleagues have described success with a "hybrid" model that uses KPD to identify a more immunologically favorable donor (although not completely free of reactivity against the donor) and then utilize desensitization techniques to facilitate transplantation.[43] This enables use of less immunosuppression for desensitization, and an increased chance of successful transplantation. This option is of great importance, given that highly sensitized recipients (PRA >80%) have had low match rates (<15%)

in KPD experience to date.[43] Blumberg and colleagues also report on their experience performing desensitization with IVIG alone in highly sensitized patients who had DSA against the donor they received through the KPD program.[44] After 22 months of follow-up, graft survival was excellent (100%) and the rate of ABMR was low (25%), considering the extent of sensitization in the patient population studied. Sharif reports another strategy successfully employed by the Hopkins transplant program, termed "rescue KPD".[45] Patients unsuccessfully desensitized against their donor are reprofiled for anti-HLA antibody after the desensitization therapy, and the incompatible pair is then entered into the KPD program in attempts to find a more compatible donor.

Transplant Center Dedication of Resources to KPD Program

The complexity of today's KPD exchanges requires participating transplant centers to allocate dedicated staff to the KPD program. KPD transplants are logistically challenging and centers wishing to participate must give thought to the infrastructure and resources needed for meaningful participation. Coordination and logistical support throughout the process is essential. Flexibility in scheduling of both donor and recipient cases is desirable, as there may be need to reschedule or rearrange on short notice in order to ensure continuity of the transplant chains.

Active participation and support from hospital administration and finance are essential, as complex insurance and financial issues may arise. A clear understanding of the benefits of transplantation over dialysis and the positive financial impact of a successful living donor transplant by hospital administrators is essential.

It has been suggested that transplant programs considering joining a KPD registry should identify a KPD Champion to lead their program, and that each KPD registry should identify mentors that have successfully implemented KPD at their own center, to provide guidance and support to new transplant centers.[15] A KPD Champion is essential in bringing together key players from both the transplant program and administration.

A transplant coordinator with hands-on experience is needed to manage the complex logistics of KPD, including entry of donors and recipients into the registry, receiving match offers, and managing logistics among transplant centers involved in a particular chain. The coordinator also maintains medical records for donor organs procured at outside centers needed for the recipient medical record, tracks the organ(s) en route to the transplant center, fields issues arising on the day of the surgery, and arranges contact between donors and recipients who wish to meet after their surgeries.

ONGOING ETHICAL ISSUES AND CONTROVERSIES

As KPD has evolved and become more complex, several ethical debates have dominated discussions about the field. The reader is referred to Chapter 4 of this textbook for a thorough discussion of these controversial issues.

CONCLUSION

Kidney paired donation is an exciting and promising solution to the current shortage of organs available for kidney transplantation. By enabling kidney transplant candidates and their willing but incompatible donors to join a KPD registry with the goal of being matched up with other pairs, KPD facilitates an increase in living donor kidney transplantation. The participation of compatible donor-recipient pairs has the potential to significantly increase the number of transplants facilitated through KPD. Benefits of living donor transplantation include superior outcomes compared to deceased donor kidney transplantation and to remaining on the deceased donor waiting list. In addition to increasing the quantity of kidney transplants, KPD offers an improvement in the quality as well, by increasing the numbers of living donor organs available to patients who might otherwise wait years on the deceased donor waiting list. KPD also provides a new opportunity for highly sensitized patients who might otherwise never receive a transplant. Movement toward one national KPD program and continued collaboration between currently participating centers may enable continued exponential growth of transplants facilitated through KPD and offers a viable strategy to address the organ shortage.

REFERENCES

1. Lysaght MJ. Maintenance dialysis population dynamics: current trends and long-term implications. J Am Soc Nephrol. 2002;13(Suppl 1):S37-40.
2. http://optn.transplant.hrsa.gov/data/. Accessed January 29, 2014.
3. http://srtr.transplant.hrsa.gov/annual_reports/2011/default.aspx. Accessed May 23, 2013.
4. Montgomery JR, Berger JC, Warren DS, et al. Outcomes of ABO-incompatible kidney transplantation in the United States. Transplantation. 2012;93(6):603-9.
5. Vo AA, Petrozzino J, Yeung K, et al. Efficacy, outcomes, and cost-effectiveness of desensitization using IVIG and Rituximab. Transplantation. 2013;95(6):852-8.
6. Archdeacon P, Chan M, Neuland C, et al. Summary of FDA antibody-mediated rejection workshop. Am J Transplant. 2011;11(5):896-906.
7. Bradley JA, Baldwin WM, Bingaman A, et al. Antibody-mediated rejection - an ounce of prevention is worth a pound of cure. Am J Transplant. 2011;11(6):1131-9.
8. Rapaport FT. The case for a living emotionally related international kidney donor exchange registry. Transplant Proc. 1986;18(3 Suppl 2):5-9.
9. Park K, Moon JI, Kim SI, et al. Exchange donor program in kidney transplantation. Transplantation. 1999;67(2):336-8.

10. de Klerk M, Witvliet MD, Haase-Kromwijk BJ, et al. Hurdles, barriers, and successes of a national living donor kidney exchange program. Transplantation. 2008;86(12):1749-53.
11. Garonzik-Wang JM, Sullivan B, Hiller JM, et al. International kidney paired donation. Transplantation. 2013;96(7):e55-6.
12. Rees MA, Kopke JE, Pelletier RP, et al. A nonsimultaneous, extended, altruistic-donor chain. N Engl J Med. 2009;360(11):1096-101.
13. Melcher ML, Leeser DB, Gritsch HA, et al. Chain transplantation: initial experience of a large multicenter program. Am J Transplant. 2012;12(9):2429-36.
14. http://www.nytimes.com/2012/02/19/health/lives-forever-linked-through-kidney-transplant-chain-124.html?pagewanted=all&_r=0. Accessed March 28, 2013.
15. Melcher ML, Blosser CD, Baxter-Lowe LA, et al. Dynamic challenges inhibiting optimal adoption of kidney paired donation: findings of a consensus conference. Am J Transplant. 2013;13(4):851-60.
16. Montgomery RA, Zachary AA, Ratner LE, et al. Clinical results from transplanting incompatible live kidney donor/recipient pairs using kidney paired donation. JAMA. 2005;294(13):1655-63.
17. Delmonico FL, Morrissey PE, Lipkowitz GS, et al. Donor kidney exchanges. Am J Transplant. 2004;4(10):1628-34.
18. Matas AJ, Garvey CA, Jacobs CL, et al. Nondirected donation of kidneys from living donors. N Engl J Med. 2000;343(6):433-6.
19. Lee YJ, Lee SU, Chung SY, et al. Clinical outcomes of multicenter domino kidney paired donation. Am J Transplant. 2009;9(10):2424-8.
20. Montgomery RA, Gentry SE, Marks WH, et al. Domino paired kidney donation: a strategy to make best use of live non-directed donation. Lancet. 2006; 368(9533):419-21.
21. Roth AE, Sönmez T, Unver MU, et al. Utilizing list exchange and nondirected donation through 'chain' paired kidney donations. Am J Transplant. 2006; 6(11):2694-705.
22. Keizer KM, de Klerk M, Haase-Kromwijk BJ, et al. The Dutch algorithm for allocation in living donor kidney exchange. Transplant Proc. 2005;37(2):589-91.
23. de Klerk M, Kal-van Gestel JA, Haase-Kromwijk BJ, et al. Eight years of outcomes of the Dutch Living Donor Kidney Exchange Program. Clin Transplant. 2011: 287-90.
24. Massie AB, Gentry SE, Montgomery RA, et al. Center-level utilization of kidney paired donation. Am J Transplant. 2013;13(5):1317-22.
25. Rees MA, Bargnesi D, Samy K, et al. Altruistic donation through the Alliance for Paired Donation. Clin Transplant. 2009:235-46.
26. Segev DL, Kucirka LM, Gentry SE, et al. Utilization and outcomes of kidney paired donation in the United States. Transplantation. 2008;86(4):502-10.
27. www.kidneyregistry.org. Accessed January 26, 2014.
28. http://transplantpro.org/wp-content/uploads/Board_11-2013_KPD_update.pdf. Accessed January 26, 2014.
29. Bingaman AW, Wright FH Jr, Kapturczak M, et al. Single-center kidney paired donation: the Methodist San Antonio experience. Am J Transplant. 2012;12(8): 2125-32.
30. http://www.organsandtissues.ca/s/english-public/living-kidney-donation/675-2. Accessed March 31, 2013.
31. Ferrari P, Fidler S, Woodroffe C, et al. Comparison of time on the deceased donor kidney waitlist versus time on the kidney paired donation registry in the Australian program. Transplant Int. 2012;25(10):1026-31.

32. Johnson RJ, Allen JE, Fuggle SV, et al. Early experience of paired living kidney donation in the United Kingdom. Transplantation. 2008;86(12):1672-7.
33. Domínguez-Gil B, de la Oliva Valentín M, Martín Escobar E, et al. Present situation of living-donor kidney transplantation in Spain and other countries: past, present and future of an excellent therapeutic option. Nefrologia. 2010;30 (Suppl 2):3-13.
34. Leeser DB, Aull MJ, Afaneh C, et al. Living donor kidney paired donation transplantation: experience as a founding member center of the National Kidney Registry. Clin Transplant. 2012;26(3):E213-22.
35. Melcher ML, Veale JL, Javaid B, et al. Kidney transplant chains amplify benefit of nondirected donors. JAMA Surg. 2013;148(2):165-9.
36. Veale J, Hil G. The National Kidney Registry: 213 transplants in three years. Clin Transplant. 2010:333-44.
37. Hurst FP, Sajjad I, Elster EA, et al. Transplantation of A2 kidneys into B and O recipients leads to reduction in waiting time: USRDS experience. Transplantation. 2010;89(11):1396-402.
38. Chen Y, Li Y, Kalbfleisch JD, et al. Graph-based optimization algorithm and software on kidney exchanges. IEEE Trans Biomed Eng. 2012;59(7):1985-91.
39. Ashlagi I, Gilchrist DS, Roth AE, et al. Nonsimultaneous chains and dominos in kidney-paired donation-revisited. Am J Transplant. 2011;11(5):984-94.
40. Gentry SE, Montgomery RA, Swihart BJ, et al. The roles of dominos and non-simultaneous chains in kidney paired donation. Am J Transplant. 2009;9(6): 1330-36.
41. Ferrari P, Fidler S, Holdsworth R, et al. High transplant rates of highly sensitized recipients with virtual crossmatching in kidney paired donation. Transplantation. 2012;94(7):744-9.
42. Cecka JM, Kucheryavaya AY, Reinsmoen NL, et al. Calculated PRA: initial results show benefits for sensitized patients and a reduction in positive crossmatches. Am J Transplant. 2011;11(4):719-24.
43. Montgomery RA, Lonze BE, Jackson AM. Using donor exchange paradigms with desensitization to enhance transplant rates among highly sensitized patients. Curr Opin Organ Transplant. 2011;16(4):439-43.
44. Blumberg JM, Gritsch HA, Reed EF, et al. Kidney paired donation in the presence of donor-specific antibodies. Kidney Int. 2013;84(5):1009-16.
45. Sharif A, Zachary AA, Hiller J, et al. Rescue kidney paired donation as emergency salvage for failed desensitization. Transplantation. 2012;93(7):e27-9.

CHAPTER 4

Ethical Issues Surrounding Opportunities to Maximize Transplantation

Mary Simmerling

ABSTRACT

The need to identify ways to maximize the number of organs available for transplantation has never been more pressing, and there are many strategies that hold unique promise for maximizing organ transplantation. These strategies include utilization of marginal donor organs, advances in minimally invasive techniques for living donor nephrectomy, and kidney paired donation. However, each strategy also poses particular ethical challenges for us to consider. This chapter discusses some of the key ethical issues that need to be attended to as we explore utilizing or expanding the use of each of these strategies as a means of maximizing organ transplantation.

INTRODUCTION

The need to identify ways to maximize the number of organs available for transplantation has never been more pressing. As of January 2014, >120,000 people were registered as waiting for deceased donor organs on the United Network for Organ Sharing organ transplant waiting list.[1] Among these 120,000 people, approximately 100,000 of them are hoping and waiting for the chance to receive one of the 11,000 deceased donor kidneys that become available each year. Of the current waiting list registrants, less than one-third can expect to receive an organ transplant in the coming year. Those left waiting for a suitable deceased donor organ face a significant risk of death, a risk that increases as they wait. It is estimated that 6,570 waiting list registrants will die this year alone because they do not get the organs they need.[1] At the present rate of transplantation, for every 79 people who are removed from this list each day because they receive an organ transplant, another 18 are removed from the list because they die waiting for one.[2] Thus, the gap between the number of organs available for transplant and the number of individuals in need of an organ transplant is not only significant, it is also deadly. And those numbers are just for the United States. The global need for organ transplants is staggering, and it is growing as the incidence of diseases such as chronic kidney disease that often lead to the need for transplantation continues to increase.[3]

The ways that we meet this need—and in some cases demand (e.g. organ trafficking, and transplant tourism)—for more organs must be carefully considered, and the complex ethical issues related to maximizing organ donation and transplantation must play an integral role in informing our decision-making. In this section, several different strategies for maximizing transplantation have been presented and discussed: the utilization of marginal, pediatric, and HCV+ deceased donor organs (Kim); advances in minimally invasive techniques for living donor nephrectomy (Watkins); and kidney paired donation (KPD) as a strategy to increase living donor kidney transplantation (Aull and Kapur). In this chapter, I discuss some of the key ethical issues that need to be attended to as we explore utilizing or expanding the use of each of these strategies as a means of maximizing organ transplantation.

UTILIZATION OF MARGINAL, PEDIATRIC, AND HCV+ DECEASED DONOR ORGANS

Kim presents compelling reasons for attempting to expand the pool of available organs by turning to organs that are already available but have heretofore gone unused or underused. Historically, the primary reason for not utilizing these organs is that they were at one time considered to be unacceptable due to the comparatively poor quality and the related increased risks and decreased benefits to the recipients compared to outcomes from standard criteria donors' (SCD) organs. Thus, the decision to utilize these organs is a decision to accept inferior outcomes for their recipients, including greater risks and fewer benefits for these recipients compared to SCD organ recipients. However, as Kim notes, the comparison to outcomes for SCD organ recipients is not the only comparison that is meaningful in this context. In fact, in many cases it may be a false choice framework, since some potential recipients may be so disadvantaged in their competition for the relatively small number of SCD organs available for transplant that there is little probability of their ever receiving an SCD organ. Understood in this way, the risks and benefits of receiving one of these organs needs also to be compared with those associated with not receiving an organ transplant at all. If the options are weighed in terms of choosing to remain on dialysis or choosing to receive an "inferior" graft, the choice to receive the inferior graft is the less risky option to take.[4-6] Pascual et al. found that patients 40 years or older, especially with diabetic nephropathy or nondiabetic disease, but a long expected waiting time for kidney transplantation, show better survival receiving an expanded criteria living donors (ECD) kidney than remaining on dialysis therapy.[6] Although they may face an increased mortality risk immediately following transplantation, the long-term mortality risk for ECD organ recipients was >50% lower for patients aged 60–74 years of age at the time of waiting list registration compared with those who remained on dialysis.[4] Although receiving one of these organs may be suboptimal compared to receiving a SCD organ, one justification for utilizing these organs is that some potential recipients have better outcomes with these organs than they otherwise would if they remained on dialysis.[5,6]

If we are to accept the use of these organs as a means of maximizing transplantation, consideration of the differential risks and benefits compared to SCD organs and not receiving a transplant at all need not only to be understood but also to be communicated clearly to the potential recipients as part of the informed consent process. Potential recipients of these organs need to be put in the best possible position to be able to evaluate the risks and benefits associated with the various options they have and supported in their decision making about which option may be the best for them. Some patients, particularly those younger than 40 years or scheduled for kidney retransplantation, should not be offered or receive an ECD kidney.[5] As Kim states, the successful utilization of these organs is predicated on carefully selecting donor traits, weighing recipient characteristics, and managing variable risk factors in order to optimize outcomes. Done in this way, and with true informed consent from recipients, the utilization of these organs may be a promising way to unburden the waiting list and reduce the cumulative negative impact of dialysis for potential recipients who would otherwise face a prolonged waiting time.

MINIMALLY INVASIVE LIVING DONOR NEPHRECTOMY

As Watkins notes, living organ donors represent the largest potential source for immediately and effectively increasing the number of organs available for transplant. Moreover, their organs are generally more desirable than organs from deceased donors. There is significant evidence that recipients of organs from living donors have an improved survival rate compared to recipients of organs from deceased donors.[7] There are several reasons for this: living donor organs are generally higher quality than deceased donor organs, living donor organs are generally better-matched to recipients than are deceased donor organs, recipients of living donor organs generally have reduced waiting times to transplantation, and the use of living organ donors allows for additional control over the timing of the transplant operation.[8] The short-term risks associated with the donation procedure are well understood and include those generally associated with anesthesia and surgery (i.e. the risk of infection or death during or after surgery, and temporary or permanent disability), as well as risks specific to organ donation, including possible damage to the remaining organ (or lobe) and possible organ failure resulting in the need for transplantation.[9] The short-term risks associated with living kidney donation have a relatively low incidence and are considered minimal beyond the risks of surgery noted above.[10] The long-term risks associated with the procedure are less well documented. In the United States, the estimated mortality rate for living kidney donors is 3.1 per 10,000 donors.[11]

Watkins presents compelling evidence that in the right surgical hands, and with the right donor, minimally invasive living donor nephrectomy may reduce risks and morbidity for donors, including less postoperative pain, faster recovery, and improvements in perioperative outcomes and other short-term measures of convalescence. These reduced risks are a major improvement in this area, and are likely to make living organ donation a more appealing option for those awaiting a transplant due to the improved safety of the surgical procedure. However, even minimally invasive living donor nephrectomy is not without risks, including operative and post-operative complications and even death. Moreover, while the short-term risks associated with the living donor surgery itself may be further decreased by using minimally invasive techniques, some of the long-term risks associated with living organ donation remain unclear and may not be impacted by the minimally invasive techniques. Also, as the acceptance criteria for living donors changes such that donors may themselves have more risk factors or "medical complexities", the reliability of existing long-term outcome data based on more stringent requirements for donation may no longer be generally applicable. The need to continue to collect data on short- and long-term donor outcomes remains as important as ever, particularly given the increased toleration for using ECD who themselves may have risk factors, such as those who are hypertensive, diabetic, or obese.[12–14]

KIDNEY PAIRED DONATION

Of all of the strategies discussed in this chapter, KPD is perhaps the most ethically complex. This is in part due to the fact that every case is different and presents its own unique set of challenges. However, one thing that is clear is that KPD has the potential to maximize transplantation by making possible transplants that would not otherwise happen. Without taking organs from the waiting list, KPD helps take people off the waiting list by transplanting them. Some of the most compelling ethical objections that have been raised against KPD are: that it is potentially more coercive because there is additional pressure not to change one's mind about donating since other people besides the intended recipient are counting on the donation; that for compatible pairs in KPD it involves an altruistically unbalanced exchange;[15] and that because living donors are disproportionately represented by Caucasians (>70%) (NKF) for reasons having to do with differences in socioeconomic status and ethnicity associated disease burdens,[16] KPD is unfair. I will discuss each of these objections in turn.

First, as I have argued elsewhere,[17] worries about the coercion of potential KPD donors can be addressed by evaluating them in the same ways and with the same rigor that all other potential living donors are evaluated. There is no reason to think that these donors should or would be evaluated differently than other potential donors who come forward for evaluation. While it is true that entering into an exchange such as KPD introduces a level of complexity and perhaps additional pressures because of the web of relationships, potential KPD donors who have agreed to be part of chains are offered the same options for changing their mind as other potential living donors. Compatible pairs who participate in KPD may in fact be less vulnerable to coercive influences than potential donors since they can decide to withdraw at any time without losing the possibility of receiving a transplant. Second, the assertion that these exchanges are "altruistically unbalanced" misses the very feature of altruism that makes it morally praiseworthy. Altruism at is essence is unselfish regard to others, sometimes at risk to oneself. As I have suggested elsewhere,[18] rather than continuing to view such altruistic motivations as suspect and their outcomes as "unbalanced", the transplant community should abandon attempts to quantify and evaluate the quality and acceptability of someone's altruism based on how much is given. Altruistic living organ donation involves unselfish giving to benefit others, with risks and costs to oneself; again, this is part of what makes it so morally praiseworthy. The transplant community must do what it can to ensure that the risks and costs associated with organ donation are minimized, reasonable, and acceptable to clinicians, donors, and recipients, regardless of whether the transplant is being done as part of a directed donation, undirected donation, exchange, or chain. Finally, there is much work to be done to address barriers to accessing KPD by non-Caucasians. However, the first step must be to identify and address barriers to accessing living organ donation by non-Caucasians. Unless and until this is resolved, participation in KPD will continue to be beyond the reach of many of the people who may stand to benefit from it the most.

CONCLUSION

Each of the strategies for maximizing transplantation discussed in this Chapter and presented in this section hold unique promise for maximizing organ transplantation. However, each strategy also poses particular ethical challenges for us to consider. The utilization of marginal, pediatric, and HCV+ deceased donor organs allows us to increase the overall number of organs available for transplantation, but introduces new risks to the recipients of those organs compared to SCD transplants. Similarly, advances in minimally invasive techniques for living donor nephrectomy offer the real potential to further minimize the risks associated with living donor nephrectomy, thereby making it a potentially safer and so also more appealing option that could lead to an increase in the overall number of living donors and so too the number of living donor organs available for transplantation. However, living organ donation is a procedure that is not without risk to the donors, including operative and postoperative complications and even death. Finally, KPD has been shown to be an effective strategy for increasing living donor kidney transplantation by identifying ways to engage willing living donor candidates in innovative exchanges and chains that allow them to obtain a compatible organ for their intended recipient to whom they could not donate (for incompatible pairs), make possible a transplant that may not otherwise happen through an organ exchange (for compatible donors), or to initiate a chain of transplants by donating an organ without an intended/specified recipient (for so-called altruistic donors). However, with the exception of altruistic donors who initiate a chain such that an organ is given to someone on waiting the list who has no potential living donor, an important ethical limitation of KPD is that one has to have a willing living donor to bring to the pool in order to get into the game. Taken together with the fact that non-Caucasians are significantly underrepresented among living donors due to socioeconomic and ethnic barriers, participation in KPD remains limited in ways that are morally problematic because they are unfairly unequal, even if they are not attributable or unique to KPD.

As we continue to explore new opportunities for maximizing organ transplantation, it is crucial that we do so with appreciation for and attention to the many ethical challenges and complexities that come with these advances. In this area of medicine where we are faced with an absolute scarce resource, we must continue to be vigilant in our quest for fairness and the possibility of equality of opportunity in access to transplantation.

REFERENCES

1. OPTN data, US Department of Health and Human Services; http://optn.transplant.hrsa.gov
2. US Kidney Disease Statistics, National Kidney and Urologic Diseases Information Clearinghouse; http://kidney.niddk.nih.gov
3. National Kidney Foundation (NKF) http://www.kidney.org/news/newsroom/factsheets/Organ-Donation-and-Transplantation-Stats.cfm
4. Wolfe RA, Ashby VB, Milford EL, et al. Comparison of mortality in all patients on dialysis, patients on dialysis awaiting transplantation and recipients of a first cadaveric transplant. N Engl J Med. 1999;341:1725-30.
5. Pascual J, Zamora J, Pirsch JD. A systematic review of kidney transplantation from expanded criteria donors. Am J Kidney Dis. 2008;52:553-86.
6. Schold JD, Meier-Kriesche HU. Which renal transplant candidates should accept marginal kidneys in exchange for a shorter waiting time on dialysis? Clin J Am Soc Nephrol. 2006;1:532-8.

7. Rager EL. The donation of human organs and the evolving capacity for transplantation: exciting developments and future prospects. N C Med J. 2004;65: 18-25.
8. Trotter JF, Wachs M, Everson GT, et al. Adult-to-adult transplantation of the right hepatic lobe from a living donor. N Engl J Med. 2002;346:1074-82.
9. American Society for Transplantation. https://www.myast.org
10. Matas AJ, Bartlett S, Leichtmen A, et al. Morbidity and mortality after living kidney donation, 1999-2001: survey of United States transplant centers. Am J Transplant. 2003;3:830-4.
11. Segev DL, Muzaale AD, Caffo BS, et al. Perioperative Mortality and Long-term Survival Following Live Kidney Donation. JAMA. 2010;303:959-66.
12. Metzger RA, Delmonico FL, Feng S, et al. Expanded criteria donors for kidney transplantation. Am J Transplant. 2003;3:114-25.
13. Stratta RJ, Rohr MS, Sundberg AK, et al. Increased kidney transplantation utilizing expanded criteria deceased organ donors with results comparable to standard criteria donor transplant. Ann Surg. 2004;239:688-95.
14. Delmonico F. Council of the Transplantation Society (2005): a report of the Amsterdam forum on the care of the live kidney donor: data and medical guidelines. Transplantation. 2005;79(Suppl 6):S53-66.
15. Ross LF, Woodle ES. Ethical issues in increasing living kidney donations by expanding kidney paired exchange programs. Transplantation. 2000;69:1539-43.
16. Bratton C, Chavin K, Baliga P. Racial disparities in organ donation and why. Curr Opin Organ Transplant. 2011;16(2):243-9.
17. Gentry SE, Segev DL, Simmerling M, et al. Expanding kidney paired donation through participation by compatible pairs. Am J Transplant. 2007;7(10):2361-70.
18. Simmerling M, Angelos P, Goldberg A, et al. Do gifts create moral obligations for recipients? Am J Bioeth. 2004;4:20-22, discussion W35-27.

2

SECTION

Considerations for Unique Patient Populations

CHAPTER 5

Considerations for the Management of Pediatric Kidney Transplant Recipients

Laurence J Belin, Anthony C Watkins

ABSTRACT

End-stage renal disease (ESRD) is a devastating diagnosis for the pediatric patient and their family. ESRD is characterized by profound metabolic abnormalities during the most formative years of life and affects the child's immune system, growth potential, and their developing sense of identity and autonomy. Kidney transplantation has the ability to provide a renewed chance at a healthy childhood, adolescence and adulthood to these young individuals. Excellent outcomes are now possible due to dramatic improvements in operative technique and modern immunosuppression. However, it is imperative that these modalities be practiced with an understanding of the unique physiologic and psychosocial makeup of the pediatric patient.

INTRODUCTION

End-stage renal disease in the pediatric population poses many unique challenges to patients, families, treating healthcare providers and systems due to unique metabolic, immunologic, neurologic, and psychosocial building blocks in comparison to the adult patient. It follows that successful renal transplantation into the pediatric recipient is not merely a matter of meticulous surgical technique in handling typically smaller donor and recipient vessels. Equally important is a rigorous attention to the intricacies of the pediatric physiology, immunology and psychology in seeking to obtain successful long-term patient and graft outcomes. An awareness of these considerations is essential to the multidisciplinary team of caregivers for these patients as, indisputably, both the survival outcomes and quality of life of a child with ESRD are dramatically improved with renal transplant relative to long-term dialysis. According to the United States Renal Data System (USRDS), 5-year patient survival probability for children undergoing kidney transplant is 91.7% compared to 78.6% for patients on hemodialysis (HD) and 80.6% for peritoneal dialysis (PD).[1] For this reason, the historic reservation in transplanting pediatric patients, including infants and small children, has given way to an enthusiasm for pre-emptive transplantation. In fact, 33% of all living donor and 13% of deceased donor renal transplants in children in the United States are now pre-emptive (NAPRTCS 2005) and 38% of patients receive a renal transplant within their first year of ESRD diagnosis. This chapter discusses the unique challenges and considerations that arise in the transplantation of a renal allograft into the pediatric patient.

ETIOLOGY OF ESRD AND CONSIDERATIONS FOR THE ABNORMAL URINARY TRACT

Between 2007–2011, the overall incidence of ESRD in children was 15.2 per million population.[1] Any discussion of issues surrounding pediatric renal transplantation must flow from an understanding of the unique causes of ESRD in children, as they are notably different from the etiologies that affect adults. The overwhelming prevalence of diabetes and hypertension seen in adult ESRD patients take a distant back seat to congenital structural abnormalities of the urinary tract, which may necessitate additional surgical correction that must be strategically timed to facilitate the successful placement and maintenance of the allograft. In 1987 the North American Pediatric Renal Transplant Cooperative Study (NAPRTCS) was initiated with an aim of collecting demographic, clinical and outcomes data on pediatric transplantation with the goal of disseminating the data to provide evidenced based practice to the pediatric renal transplant community. Obstructive uropathy and renal dysplasia together make up nearly a third of cases of ESRD in children in the NAPRTCS registry with glomerular disorders comprising an additional 23%. Specifically, focal segmental glomerular sclerosis (FSGS) comprises 11.7% of primary diagnoses and represents the leading cause of acquired kidney disease in children.[2] As is the case in the adult population, the etiology of ESRD in children demonstrates racial variability, with FSGS accounting for a quarter of ESRD in black recipients, while the congenital pathologies represent a third of cases in whites and Hispanics.

Major congenital urologic abnormalities are often present in children with ESRD and necessitate adjunctive surgical procedures in up to 40% of potential graft recipients.[3] These may include a range of interventions from simple intermittent catheterization to major surgery including bladder augmentation and reconstruction of urethral sphincter mechanisms. Transplant graft survival is superior when abnormalities are confined to the upper urinary tract proximal and/or including the ureterovesical junction (UVJ). These abnormalities are more intrinsic to the native kidneys and ureters as opposed to the lower abnormalities of the bladder, sphincter and urethra. If uncorrected, lower congenital uropathies threaten graft survival by compromising the ability of the lower urinary tract to store and empty urine. The resulting obstructive uropathy results in ischemia, nephron destruction and graft necrosis. The clinician's chief concern when confronted with evaluating a potential transplant candidate is to determine whether the renal pathology present requires additional surgical correction beyond isolated transplantation. This basic workup should include a careful history and physical examination, urine studies including urinalysis, 24-h urine protein, urine gram stain and culture, renal and ureteral ultrasound. Furthermore, when suspicion of lower tract abnormalities is low, noninvasive flow studies are indicated prior to proceeding with transplantation. Patients with suspicious findings or known congenital disorders such as posterior urethral valves, neurogenic bladder, severe ureterocele, bladder extrophy, and cloacal abnormalities require additional evaluation. For these patients, workup includes a voiding cystourethrogram, CT scans to evaluate renal size, and contrast evaluation of upper and lower urinary tracts for structure, obstruction and the presence of reflux. Patients with lower urinary tract abnormalities require urodynamic testing and direct visualization of bladder and ureteral orifices with cystoscopy.

Surgical correction of congenital lower tract abnormalities seeks to restore an adequate urinary reservoir at low pressure, competent urethral control mechanisms capable of continence, and a patent passageway for complete bladder evacuation via voiding or catheterization. This may involve augmentation cystoplasty and/or reconstruction of urethral sphincter mechanisms. The guiding principle is to complete reconstruction of the lower urinary tract prior to transplantation and the subsequent immunosuppressed state.

Furthermore, in cases of severe cystic parenchymal disease, large Wilm's tumor, or massive hamartoma, the native kidney's mass effect may preclude transplant prior to native nephrectomy. Native kidney stasis, reflux, and pre-existing urologic stomas may be an infectious source for florid sepsis in a setting of post-transplant immunosuppression. Thus, indications for pretransplant nephrectomy or nephroureterectomy include removal of a source of stasis and infection, large size, malignancy, renin-sensitive hypertension refractory to pharmacologic control, and severe protein and water wasting.[3]

In summary, the infant or child awaiting a renal transplant is approached with the assumption that placement of the renal allograft is the end event in a sequence of surgical correction necessary to restore both the renal filtering and evacuating mechanisms. The transplant surgeon and patient should proceed to the operating room for renal transplant only when all other urologic abnormalities are either ruled out, corrected, or a clear plan has been implemented for repair in conjunction with colleagues from urologic surgery.

DETERMINANTS OF OUTCOME IN THE PEDIATRIC POPULATION

Graft Survival

The past two decades have demonstrated substantial improvement in pediatric transplant outcomes, and it is now not uncommon for grafts to survive well past a decade. An understanding of factors associated with short- and long-term allograft function is of increasing importance and is an active area of investigation. Understanding the mechanisms that positively influence graft survival provides surgeons and nephrologists with evidence-based practice that will allow for more and more children to live into adulthood with functioning kidneys.

Several large studies have sought to define the major risk factors that influence pediatric renal transplant survival. According to an analysis of the United Network for Organ Sharing (UNOS) registry between 1987–1998, living donor transplants demonstrate superior 1-year graft survival (93%) compared to deceased donor (85%) and this difference persists at 5 years (80% vs 75%, respectively).[4] The superior outcome of living donor grafts relative to deceased donor grafts has been echoed by other series and is now well-established although the benefit is narrowing.

Utilizing follow-up data on >8,000 pediatric renal transplants in the UNOS registry, Gjertson et al. found the most dominant factor attributable to beneficial variation in short-term outcomes was the use of maintenance immunosuppression, cyclosporine (CsA), or tacrolimus (Prograf).[4] Similarly, Ellis et al. examined the NARPTCS registry entries between 1987–1993 and identified a cohort of patients <12 years of age at transplant for whom 10-year follow-up data were available.[5] A univariate analysis of these 1903 patients found that, in comparison to patients with a functioning graft at 10-year post-transplant, patients with a failed transplant prior to this time tended to be older, female, non-Caucasian, and had a primary diagnosis of FSGS. Furthermore, failure was more often seen with deceased donor transplants from younger donors, HLA mismatches, pretransplant HD, history of prior transplant, and delayed graft function (DGF). Failed transplant recipients were also less likely to receive prednisone, CsA and azathioprine in the first month of post-transplant. Taken together, these data on short- and long-term outcomes highlight the importance of pre-emptive transplant, where possible, maintenance immunosuppression, and the superiority of well-matched living donor grafts.

The causes of graft failure in pediatric recipients are distinctly different than that seen most frequently in the adult transplant literature. The leading cause of graft loss in children is due to chronic rejection, responsible for up to a third of cases. The second leading cause of graft failure in children is due to technical causes and reflects the difficulty of creating a tension-free and patent vascular anastomosis between diminutive recipient and vessels and donor organs. Among these technical failures, roughly 10% of graft losses are due to vascular thrombosis.[6] Technical complications are particularly true among children of younger age. Among recipients <2 years of age receiving a living donor transplant, technical causes of graft loss are the etiology behind 33% of failure of which 24% are due to primary vascular thrombosis. Comparatively, graft thrombosis in adults is a rare event. In addition, the occurrence of postoperative acute tubular necrosis (ATN) in pediatric transplant recipients appears to have a considerable detrimental effect on outcome and is a major independent risk factor for graft failure in infants. ATN results in a 20–35% inferior graft survival at all time points following transplantation. Thus, in addition to ideal donor and recipient characteristics, meticulous surgical technique is also paramount in order to avoid technical complication and ATN, thereby optimizing the likelihood of long-term graft function.

Graft Rejection

With advancements in immunosuppressive regimens, annual rejection rates have declined over time; however, rejection remains the single greatest threat to graft viability. In an outcomes report of the NARPTCS representing 11,603 pediatric recipient kidney transplants between 1987–2010, immunologic mediated graft loss was the number one cause of graft failure.[2] The cumulative 1-year acute rejection rate between 2004–2010 was 15% in the NARPTCS. Of these, 35.3% were due to chronic rejection, 13.2% due to acute rejection, and 1.9% resulting from hyperacute rejection. Importantly, living donors had lower rates of rejection in comparison to deceased donors (8.6 vs 16.6%). Additional factors associated with acute rejection included age of transplant >12 years of age, black race, and DGF.

There is a paucity of literature on the incidence, prognosis and optimal therapy for acute antibody-mediated rejection (AMR) in children. AMR is characterized by allograft dysfunction in the setting of donor-specific antibodies (DSA) and biopsy proven evidence of inflammation. AMR may occur early or late post-transplant and may have dire consequences for the graft, as it is a steroid resistant and progressive entity. The etiology of AMR involves multiple facets of the immune system including the activation of helper T cells, memory B cells and antibody production, thus effective treatment must address each of these components. Typical treatment courses in adult patients include intravenous immunoglobulin (IVIG), plasmapheresis and plasma exchange. Recently, the use of the monoclonal anti-CD20 agent rituximab has been added to the treatment of refractory cases. The use of these modalities in children is reported in several small series in the literature with encouraging results. One single center 5-year experience with 86 pediatric kidney transplants demonstrated an AMR rate of 7.7%.[7] All patients were treated with high dose steroids and IVIG initially which resulted in resolution of graft function in three, the remainder required plasmapheresis and three resistant patients received rituximab. Two of these patients were refractory to all treatment and lost their grafts. A second series of 58 children demonstrated AMR in 3 (5.2%) and reported treatment success with the utilization the proteasome inhibitor bortezomib in two patients.[8] This agent has demonstrated activity against mature plasma cells, the primary cell involved in DSA production, and a few case reports in adult transplant patients have demonstrated beneficial effects in the treatment of AMR.

Empiric treatment of AMR in pediatric recipients is typically based on clinical condition and not protocoled at most institutions. The development of evidence-based treatment protocols are desperately needed as 1-year graft survival in the face of AMR ranges from 62% to 71% in retrospective series. In the absence of larger randomized trials, early diagnosis and multimodal treatment is of paramount importance in the treatment of AMR. Present data support the use of high-dose steroids to suppress immune response, IVIG, and plasmapheresis to remove circulating antibodies and consideration of rituximab or bortezomib for their cytotoxic effect on B cells.

DEVELOPMENTAL PHARMACOLOGY AND IMMUNOSUPPRESSION STRATEGIES IN THE PEDIATRIC PATIENT

Immunosuppressive regimens and therapeutic windows for pediatric transplant patients have mostly been extrapolated from data and experience with adult immunosuppressive pharmacokinetics. Studies examining therapeutic efficacy and toxicity in pediatric populations are few and, in fact, multiple chronic immunosuppressive medications, including CsA, prednisone, and azathioprine are not FDA approved for pediatric use. Yet it is well-established that there exist many variations in the infant, pediatric, and adolescent patients in the four cornerstones of pharmacokinetics: absorption, distribution, metabolism and elimination.

Gastrointestinal absorption is a pH-dependent process that relies on gastric and intestinal motility as well as mucosal integrity, all of which vary in pediatric patients from their adult norms. In infants and children <3 years old, a relatively immature and achlorhydric gastric mucosa results in decreased absorption of medications requiring acidic environments. Furthermore, gastric and intestinal motility is erratic in pediatric patients, and ranges with age, from sluggish in neonates to hypermotile in infancy and adolescence.

After variable absorption of immunosuppressive medications, important age-related differences are present in body composition of water and fat that significantly affect pharmacokinetics. The neonate possesses a significantly elevated total and extracellular body water component that declines to normal by 9 months of age. Fat composition decreases from infancy to childhood only to increase again by adolescence at which time gender differences are present. Circulating plasma protein levels are typically lower in the neonate, resulting in less drug binding interactions and a greater free fraction of available drug per given dose.[9]

Drug metabolism is also associated with age and gender variations. Levels of cytochrome P450 enzymes are typically low in the neonate but rise above adult levels in childhood. Furthermore, the metabolic pathways responsible for methylation, sulfation, acetylation and conjugation vary in children, which may have an end result of impeding drug delivery to target organs. Finally, renal elimination is impaired in infancy with a low GFR and capacity for tubular excretion, which must be accounted for when considering the drug clearance capacity of an infant transplant patient.

Modern immunosuppression strategies for pediatric recipients are typically weight based polyclonal (antithymocyte globulin) or monoclonal anti-IL2R (basiliximab, daclizumab) antibody based induction regimens with a calcineurin inhibitor (CNI) based maintenance protocol. Up to half of patients are receiving induction therapy. This typically includes tacrolimus or CsA used in conjunction with mycophenolate mofetil or azathioprine and prednisone.

Due to the particular sensitivity of infants and children with the double insult of ESRD and immunosuppression to growth delay, modern protocols make a concerted emphasis at steroid sparing when possible. Steroid withdrawal may be done early (~1 week post-transplant in a setting of induction antibody therapy) or later when allograft function is deemed stable at 1-year post-transplant. In the above NAPRTC analysis, only 48.8% of patients were using steroids at 1-month postoperatively in 2009. The largest study examining the effect of early steroid withdrawal (~1 week post-transplant) on the longitudinal growth of pediatric renal transplant patients was the TWIST study, a randomized two-arm multicenter study including 196 participants from Europe, South Africa and Israel.[10] At 6 months of follow-up, this trial demonstrated a significant improvement in height standard deviation among steroid withdrawal (induction with four days of steroid taper), which was accompanied by favorable changes in lipid and triglyceride profiles as well as glycemic control. Importantly, rejection rates were low in both arms (10.2% steroid arm vs 7.1% steroid withdrawal) and graft survival and function were equivalent at 6-month post-transplant. Longer-term follow-up is pending but in the short term, steroid withdrawal based regimens appear safe and no less efficacious.

The CNIs have dramatically improved short-term graft survival and acute rejection rates in both adult and pediatric renal transplantation since their introduction in the 1980s; however, their chronic use has a significant capacity for nephrotoxicity. This is of particular concern in pediatric kidney transplantation due to the considerable number of life years under immunosuppression ahead of the young patient. Increasingly, there has been a push to reduce exposure to CNIs due to the delicate balance between benefit and graft nephrotoxicity seen with tacrolimus and CsA. Complete CsA avoidance has been associated with a 10–20% increase in acute rejection episodes in some studies, so present enthusiasm is for finding strategies that allow for the minimization of CNI use.[11] One such strategy is the addition of mammalian target of rapamycin (mTOR) inhibitors, rapamycin, sirolimus and everolimus, to maintenance regimens. Although large controlled trials are lacking, multiple prospective single-arm studies have demonstrated efficacy of mTOR inhibitors with reduced CNI in pediatric kidney transplant.[12] As maintenance therapy, the switch from standard CNI-based therapy to mTOR with low-dose CNI or CNI-free regimens effectively prevent rejection and have a low risk of infectious complications. Advocates of mTOR-based regimens recommend an early (6-month post-transplant) conversion to mTOR/CNI-minimized regimens when not prohibited by declining graft function in order to maximize the benefit to the graft. Taken together, steroid withdrawal and the minimization of CNI-based maintenance regimens appear to be safe, efficacious, and advisable among children of low immunologic risk.

ADULT SIZE AND EXPANDING THE DONOR POOL

It is well-established that living donor grafts demonstrate superior survival than deceased donors in children. In comparison to adults, pediatric recipients receive a disproportionate number of living donor organs due to the availability and emotional investment of parents and family as potential donors. In 2001, living donation accounted for 61% of transplanted organs captured by the NAPRTCS with 40% of those coming from parents. This proportion has leveled off somewhat in recent years but nonrelated living donation is on the rise. With the advent and implementation of modern immunosuppression regimens, the survival benefit between living donation and deceased donation is narrowing in pediatric transplantation. Although historically used with reservation, deceased donor transplants into children are resulting in satisfactory patient and graft short- and long-term outcomes. At present, however, the worst outcomes are to be expected when the youngest recipient age groups receive deceased donor grafts from pediatric donors.

Adult size kidneys (ASKs) have been shown to provide excellent long-term outcomes in infants and children provided ATN is avoided. The ASK transplanted into the pediatric patient is particularly prone to the occurrence of ATN due to the small blood volume and cardiac output of the recipient infant or child being inadequate to optimally perfuse the larger mass of the adult kidney. In even the most optimal of circumstances, it is estimated that the infant can only provide two-thirds of the original blood flow seen by the adult kidney. As a result, the newly transplanted adult kidney is at great risk for hypoperfusion, ischemia and ATN. This scenario may be avoided with aggressive fluids and salt loading to maintain a SBP >95th percentile for age. One single center study examined their experience with 45 consecutive recipients weighing <15 kg.[13] Among recipients receiving ASKs, four had an occurrence of ATN and all subsequently had acute rejection episodes, whereas none of the 32 ASKs without ATN went on to have an episode of acute rejection. Interestingly at 3 years post-transplantation, ASKs with ATN had a significantly higher baseline serum creatinine (mean 1.5 vs 0.9 mg/dL). Long-term graft survival was superior among recipients with ASKs without ATN relative to those with ATN and this was true in both living donors and cadaveric donors. To this point, a secondary analysis in the above study examined living donor ASK without ATN transplanted into pediatric recipients in the UNOS registry. The graft half-life of a living donor ASK without ATN transplanted into children ages 0–5 was found to be equivalent or better than that of a graft from an HLA identical sibling in adult age groups.

In adult renal transplantation, the push to expand the eligible donor pool has led to encouraging new avenues for transplantation, specifically the use of donation after cardiac death (DCD) kidneys and en-bloc renal transplants from small pediatric donors. It is worth mentioning the limited literature describing the use of these organs in pediatric recipients. In adults, DCD kidneys have demonstrated graft and patient survival comparable to that seen with donation after brain death (DBD). The experience describing DCD kidneys in children is sparse and typically limited by small sample sizes. The largest series to date describes 137 pediatric recipients of DCD kidneys between 1994 and 2010 registered with the Scientific Registry of Transplant Recipients and compared outcomes with 6059 DBD kidney recipients during the same time period.[14] Recipients of DCD kidneys had a significantly higher rate of DGF relative to DBD recipients (22% vs 12.3%) and a twofold increase in graft loss was evident among DCD recipients at and beyond 4 years post-transplant. However, more experience is needed with DCD donors in children. At present they are a viable option to expand the donor pool for children awaiting transplant and data in adults suggest excellent outcomes are possible.

Adult transplant literature has demonstrated equivalent to superior long-term survival of en-bloc pediatric allografts from small donors as compared to solitary pediatric kidneys.[15] The literature on the use of these grafts in pediatric transplantation is again limited; however, several small case series exist describing the use of en-bloc grafts in children with good short-term outcomes. The earliest of these described the use of en-bloc kidneys from small donors into three pediatric recipients with no thrombotic complications; rejection or graft loss and all grafts demonstrated increase in longitudinal size measured by ultrasound.[16] A 2012 single institution series summarized 8 en-bloc transplantations into pediatric recipients over 5 years.[17] In this series, three patients had perioperative complications which included ATN, graft hematoma, and allograft thrombosis of one of the en-bloc kidneys necessitating nephrectomy while the sister kidney was viable and left in situ. Despite these complications, no patient experienced DGF, all grafts demonstrated increased renal length on follow-up ultrasound and median serum creatinine at follow-up was 0.67 mg/dL. One patient experienced acute humoral rejection. The authors of this study concluded that the use of en-bloc kidneys from young donors is safe with an acceptable complication risk, highlighting the lack of vascular thrombosis among the grafts. Both studies demonstrate one benefit of the use of en-bloc kidneys in pediatric recipients is the ability of the graft to grow with the child, increasing GFR over time. Providing these small kidneys preferentially to pediatric recipients rather than adults also negates concerns for donor/recipient size discrepancies and the threat of hyperperfusion injury to the graft. Whether these theoretical assumptions prove true and clinically relevant in larger trials will require more experience. Certainly, further longitudinal and larger studies are required before en-bloc pediatric grafts transplanted into pediatric recipients can be recommended but the existing case reports and series are generally encouraging. At present this approach is underutilized and further experience will facilitate greater technical expertise in transplanting these small kidneys, improving outcomes, and providing an avenue to expand the available donor pool and reduce wait times for pediatric recipients.

CAUSES OF MORBIDITY AND MORTALITY IN PEDIATRIC KIDNEY TRANSPLANT RECIPIENTS

The leading causes of death among transplanted children are secondary to infectious causes followed by, cardiovascular mortality, and malignancy. The largest study examining mortality in children after renal transplantation looked at nearly 2,500 patients in the NAPRTCS registry for approximately 5,500 patient-years post-transplantation and determined the annual death rate to be 24.8 per 1,000 patient years.[18] Mortality was highest among recipients <1 year old at transplant and decreased steadily with age to a nadir of 4.5% in adolescents. Interestingly, the greater the concordance between young donor and recipient age, the higher likelihood of mortality in the recipient. Cadaver-donor source was associated with a significantly higher mortality rate (6.7%) than living donor (4%), as was the presence of ATN or graft failure within 30 days of operation.

As with their adult counterparts, infants and children with ESRD are at heightened risk for infectious complications due to their underlying chronic disease, nutritional and growth deficits, immunosuppressed state, and frequent need for hospitalization. Unlike adults, however, the pediatric patient has unique characteristics that make them particularly prone to infection, including a relative lack of exposure to pathogens and consequent lack of pre-existing immunity. As such, pediatric renal transplant patients have a higher risk of infection than adult transplant patients.

Among children with ESRD, the highest risk for infectious mortality is faced by the youngest patients. The United States Renal Data System (USRDS) notes recent mortality rates attributable to infection of 19.1 per 1,000 patient among ages 0–9, compared to 2.9 and 2.2 per 1,000 patient years among children age 10–14 and 15–19, respectively.[1] Relative to children on dialysis, transplantation results in decreased risk for infectious mortality. Septic mortality among children on HD and PD are similar, at approximately 10.0 per 1,000 patient years. This number is three times higher than the infectious mortality rate of children with a renal transplant (USRDS 2013[19]) although infection remains the leading cause of death in this population, representing the cause of death in 30% of cases. Infections in the pediatric renal transplant recipient are typically most severe and life-threatening when immunosuppression is highest, during the 6-month perioperative period. Infections within the first month of transplant are characterized by the typical nosocomial infections of the urinary tract, wound and line infections, and pneumonias, as well as donor derived and recipient opportunistic infections with colonizing organisms.

Beyond the immediate post-transplant period, infections are now the number one cause of hospitalization during the first 2 years post-transplant as well, with numbers double that of acute rejection.[20] Infection-associated hospitalizations during 2 years post-transplant are significantly associated with antibody induction, ATN, age <2 year at transplant, greater than five pretransplant transfusions, and a non-pre-emptive transplant in one study of the NARPTCS.[21] Infectious hospitalizations are evenly split between viral and bacterial diseases and typically include lower and upper urinary tract infection, cytomegalovirus (CMV) and BK graft nephropathy, and both viral and bacterial pneumonias. The potential sources are many and varied and include both community and hospital acquired sources, latent viral infections, and opportunistic organisms. Donor derived infections may include bacterial infections with *Staphylococcus, Streptococcus pneumoniae, Escherichia coli,* and *Candida* species. The recipient is also at heightened risk for antimicrobial resistant organisms with which they may have been colonized preoperatively. These include methicillin-resistant *Staphylococcus aureus*, vancomycin-resistant *Enterococcus*, and resistant strains of *Candida, Aspergillus* and *Clostridium*. Disseminated fungal infections including the mycoses (histoplasmosis, coccidioidomycosis, cryptococcus) may gain entrance through venous or bladder cannulation and may be quite severe and require prolonged therapy.

The most significant pathogen in pediatric renal transplant, as with adult, is CMV. Risk factors for viral infection identified in an analysis of pediatric recipients in the USRDS include age <18 and donor CMV positive status.[22] Pretransplant CMV positive status in the recipient was associated with decreased risk, likely reflecting pretransplant exposure and immune response against the virus.

Treatment of invasive infections in pediatric renal transplant begins with prophylaxis. Peri- and postoperative antibiotics with a broad-spectrum cephalosporin or fluoroquinolone is standard at most centers. Prophylaxis against *Pneumocystis jiroveci* and the common causative organisms of urinary tract infection is accomplished with daily trimethoprim and sulfamethoxazole, typically for 6 months postoperatively. Ganciclovir is used both prophylactically and therapeutically against CMV infection. Treatment of invasive infections in the pediatric recipient is a delicate balance between reducing immunosuppression to allow for enough immune reconstitution to allow the host response to assist systemic antimicrobials in clearing the infection without precipitating graft rejection. It is imperative to treat in an inpatient setting and let culture results guide therapy. Monitoring of graft function, including biopsy where necessary, is advisable under lightened immunosuppression.

Of particular concern in pediatric transplant recipients is vaccination status as influenza and pneumococcal infections are an important preventable cause of morbidity and hospitalization. Unfortunately, vaccination rates for children with functioning renal transplants are half of those of adult counterparts in the 2013 USRDS.[19] Furthermore, transplant recipients demonstrate lower vaccination rates than children on HD. Since hospitalizations due to influenza and pneumococcal pneumonia are frequent, especially among younger patients, this is an important area for preventive awareness and improvement. In summary, infections may be catastrophic among renal transplant patients, and children are even more at risk. An aggressive approach must be taken toward ensuring appropriate vaccination, prophylaxis, and early treatment upon clinical suspicion of invasive infection.

Second only to infection, cardiovascular disease accounts for 40–50% of all deaths among pediatric patients with ESRD. In fact, children afflicted with ESRD possess an age-adjusted 700-fold increased risk of cardiac death compared to healthy children. Black race and HD have been identified as risk factors imposing heightened risk. The pathophysiology in children poorly understood but the mechanism appears to be distinct from the typical atherosclerotic plaque formation seen in adult patients. Instead, it is believed that uremia predisposes to endothelial cell dysfunction which ultimately results in arterial medial calcification, consequent arterial wall thickening and compensatory left ventricular wall hypertrophy, conduction abnormalities and both coronary and small vessel disease. Interestingly, despite the fact that these proposed mechanisms evolve over years, the highest risk of myocardial infarction appears to be in children <5 years. It has been suggested that vulnerability in this age group is instead due to a heightened susceptibility to uremia, fluid shifts, and anemia characteristic of ESRD.

Renal transplantation appears to confer a protective effect and decrease cardiovascular mortality in children with ESRD. A large retrospective observational study of the USRDS analyzed 1380 deaths from 1990 to 1996 among children who started ESRD therapy and died before the age of 30.[23] In this cohort, cardiac deaths occurred in 34% of dialysis patients of black race and 25% of white patients. This number dropped to 11% of black transplant recipients and 9% of white recipients. All in all, children with a functioning graft had a 78% reduced risk of cardiac mortality in this study. The odds ratio for cardiac death before the age of 30 in pediatric patients with ESRD who received a transplant was 0.22 relative to dialysis patients.

It is important to note, however, that despite an impressive risk reduction, transplant patients still maintain a markedly higher risk of cardiac death than the general population. Factors that may play a role in this persistence is the age of onset of ESRD and the length of time on renal replacement therapy prior to obtaining a functioning graft. Presently, there are no studies in the literature to examining whether transplantation results in remodeling and resolution of existing left ventricular hypertrophy from years of uremia. Similarly, pretransplant ESRD children on PD are known to have elevations in lipoprotein A, cholesterol and LDL, and these unfavorable lipid profiles are known to persist post-transplantation.[24] Furthermore, children with ESRD who are successfully transplanted are characterized by other persistent cardiac risk factors including hypertension, and the use of steroids and tacrolimus, which are known lipogenic agents in the transplant patient.

MALIGNANCY

The risk of any-cancer development is estimated to be twofold higher in recipients of solid organ transplants relative to the general population due, in part, to a chronic immunosuppressed state. Among pediatric recipients of kidney transplant, approximately 10% of all deaths are related to cancer. The majority of these cases incident in childhood and adolescence are secondary to post-transplant lymphoproliferative disorder (PTLD). PTLD describes a category of lymphoid malignancies that represent an end stage of events whose origin has been traced to Epstein-Barr infection of B cells. Immunocompetent patients can elicit a robust T-cell response against infected cells; however, in the immunosuppressed transplant patient, malignant transformation and expansion may result. Pediatric kidney transplant patients are at even greater risk of PTLD than their adult counterparts. In the recent USRDS annual data report, the cumulative incidence of PTLD within 36 months of transplant was 1.54% among pediatric patients compared to 0.45% among adults, a threefold increase in incident cases.[19]

Factors associated with increased risk of PTLD are EBV seronegative status at transplantation (fourfold increased risk), CMV seronegative status (twofold increased risk), complete HLA-DR mismatch, and age at transplant, with younger patients at higher risk.[25] Furthermore, induction therapy with thymoglobulin and OKT3 are associated with an increased risk of PTLD leading to their conservative use or complete omission in modern protocols.[26] The data on individual maintenance agents are derived from retrospective series and generally inconclusive.

In adult transplant recipients, the risk of cancer is not limited to PTLD as the immunosuppressed state may provide fertile ground for other cancers as well. The common theme among the leading malignancies after solid organ transplant is a putative infectious origin: PTLD (EBV), Kaposi's sarcoma (HHV-8), hepatocellular carcinoma (HBV and HCV), and the human papillomavirus related epithelial cancers predominate. The incidence of *Helicobacter pylori* associated gastric cancer is elevated as well. In addition to these cancers, adult solid organ transplant (SOT) patients are at elevated risk for renal and lung malignancies.

While the majority of cancer among pediatric transplant patients is PTLD, with improving long-term graft and patient survival in recent years, these children are surviving into adulthood at which time they face the risk of these other malignancies. The risk for squamous and basal cell carcinomas approach 15% at 15 years post-transplantation, although rarely in childhood, and is treated with surgery with or without a reduction in immunosuppression. Pediatric kidney transplant patients have been reported to have a 0.6% chance of renal cell carcinoma. De novo kidney cancer typically occurs in the native kidneys and risk is highest (approximately 15-fold greater than general population) in youngest patients.[27] Most cases are localized and effectively treated with partial or total native nephrectomy.

Finally, a word should be said about recurrence of pretransplant cancer. Children treated with nephrectomy and/or chemotherapy for Wilm's tumor may develop ESRD. Additionally, ESRD in children may develop as sequelae of bone marrow transplant for pediatric leukemia. Though lacking solid evidence, common practice is to defer renal transplantation for 2 years after definitive cancer therapy to provide a period of surveillance for recurrent disease.

While a discussion of the individual treatment options for each of the cancer diagnoses is outside the reach of this chapter, the obvious consideration is the balance between avoiding graft rejection while allowing enough immune reconstitution to aid in tumor surveillance and destruction. The mainstay in treatment for PTLD is a reduction in immunosuppression that has been shown to induce complete remission in up to 50% of patients.[28] Prognosis is fair for these patients with 2-year overall survival in the literature ranging from 70% to 83%. Favorable prognostic factors include younger age, CD20 expression, early occurrence (<1 year after transplant) and good response to first-line treatment.

If reduction in immunosuppressive drugs is not possible due to evidence of graft rejection or proving insufficient to control disease, rituximab is added in CD-20 positive disease as monotherapy or in combination with systemic chemotherapy. The use of the mTOR inhibitors rapamycin and sirolimus as part of immunosuppression is also advocated due to proposed antitumor activity in PTLD as well as other mTOR pathway activated tumors such as squamous cell, post-transplant smooth muscle spindle tumors, and Kaposi's sarcoma.[29]

In the absence of any validated laboratory or screening parameters for malignancy in pediatric recipients of renal transplants, surveillance and early recognition must rely on physical examination with an emphasis on dermatologic, gynecologic, and ano-genital examinations to detect premalignant or early malignant lesions. If native kidneys remain in situ, periodic ultrasound should be obtained to detect suspicious renal lesions.

GROWTH DELAY IN THE PEDIATRIC PATIENT WITH ESRD

End-stage renal disease in children results in growth retardation via several proposed mechanisms, including chronic acidosis, renal osteodystrophy resulting from primary secondary hyperparathyroidism, insufficient caloric intake, and perturbations in the growth hormone/insulin like growth factor axis. This has lead to the use of recombinant growth factor in children with ESRD as a temporizing measure but catch up growth and normal adult growth is rarely observed. Even following transplant, immunosuppression medications, including corticosteroids, provide an obstacle to the recipient obtaining the growth potential of their healthier peers. Height deficits are typically greater for males than females and for younger patients and those with a history of prior transplant.[2]

Renal transplantation's rescue effect on growth is sporadic and incomplete. To date, the most informative analysis examined 20 years of growth data collected by the NAPRTCS.[30] At the time of transplantation, this population had a mean height deficit of 1.75 standard deviations below age and sex-adjusted height level. Only children <6 years of age at transplant demonstrated growth acceleration following transplant; however, it was precisely these youngest patients who had the greatest degree of growth retardation at baseline with Z scores of –2.0 or greater. The impact of chronic steroid use on growth was also demonstrated by this data. Complete steroid avoidance resulted in a degree of catch up growth within 3 years of transplantation; however, alternating day regimens resulted in no such growth and daily regimens demonstrated a gradual progressive decline in Z score as far out as 5 years. The use of recombinant GH resulted in a modest Z score improvements of +0.5 standard deviations after 5 years of use.

PSYCHOSOCIAL CONSIDERATIONS

A growing body of literature suggests that children transplanted as adolescents have an increased risk of graft loss, late acute rejection, and incomplete resolution of rejection episodes compared to children transplanted at younger age groups. This may be due, in part, to the unique and evolving psychosocial motivations of the child and adolescent recipient of SOT, which may be at odds with the high level of investment and cooperation necessary for the care of their transplanted organ. In a study among pediatric heart transplant patients surviving >1 year, 10-year survival in patients transplanted as an adolescent was found to be 63%, whereas 10-year survival was 69% among children age 1–10, and 77% in infants <1 year.[31] While the reasons behind inferior survival among adolescent patients relative to their younger peers are multifactorial and both physiologic and pharmacokinetic factors may be involved, it has been suggested that the ability of an adolescent patient to adhere to demanding and chronic immunosuppressive treatment and physician follow-up is challenged by the dynamic psychosocial milieu of that age group. During this period, the usual push for autonomy and a developing self-identify is at odds with respect for authority, and adult institutions including medical staff, caregivers, and treatments. Compounding these stresses, the transplant adolescent has spent much or all of his or her life living with chronic disease, and potential developmental and physical delays that aggravate body image insecurities characteristic of their age group.[9] This perfect storm may be a recipe for immunosuppressant noncompliance and it is essential that treating physicians include a general pediatrician or child and adolescent psychiatrist who is uniquely tuned in to these issues and provides the patient with a platform to express and handle their turmoil. Care for the pediatric transplant recipient must go beyond the surgeon and nephrologist and engage family and other psychosocial support services as well to ensure that the child is utilizing healthy coping mechanisms with their disease, expressing their frustrations and an active participant in their treatment program.

RETRANSPLANTATION

With an estimated 5-year patient survival of 96% and a 5-year graft survival of 85% for LDs and 75% for DDs, pediatric recipients of kidney transplantation frequently have a life expectancy that exceeds their graft. While not unique to pediatric transplant, the issue of retransplantation is encountered more frequently in children who, in the best of circumstances, have more life-years ahead of them than their adult counterparts and thus frequently become candidates for retransplantation. A 2003 survey examining pediatric recipients surviving into adulthood found that nearly half had undergone retransplantation.[32] Multiple issues arise in this scenario, including the risk of sensitization from the first transplant negatively impacting the subsequent graft, thus raising questions regarding the optimal sequence of donor types when only one living donor is available. Historical strategy encouraged the use of a living donor first due to their superior longevity. However, a recent observational study of nearly 15,000 pediatric recipients including 1663 retransplants in the SRTS revealed that living donor grafts had longer survival than deceased donor both as first and second transplants.[33] Additionally, this finding held true whether a living donor as second transplant succeeded a prior living donor or deceased donor graft. Of note, however, was the finding that the cumulative graft life of combined deceased donor and living donor retransplants was similar regardless of the order of transplantation. This suggests that an index deceased donor kidney transplant in pediatric recipients does not negatively impact the expected survival of a later living donor transplant. These data are encouraging for the prospect of retransplantation as more and more first deceased donor grafts are being offered to pediatric recipients in light of UNOS recent Share-35 allocations.

CONCLUSION

Truly, the impact of ESRD upon an infant or child is potentially unparalleled in its complexity and capacity for devastation. Renal failure is characterized by profound metabolic abnormalities during the most formative years in the life of a human being. End-stage renal disease's touch corrupts everything from the child's immune system and growth potential to their developing sense of identity and autonomy. The miracle of renal transplantation has given the gift of a renewed chance at a healthy childhood, adolescence and adulthood to these young individuals. Excellent outcomes are now made possible by dramatic improvements in operative technique and modern immunosuppression. However, it is imperative that these modalities be practiced with an understanding of the unique physiologic and psychosocial makeup of the pediatric patient. No greater is the awe of organ transplantation evident than in the successful treatment of a child with ESRD culminating in the growth of an adult living free of it.

REFERENCES

1. Collins AJ, Foley RN, Chavers B, et al. United States Renal Data System 2011 Annual Data Report: atlas of chronic kidney disease & end-stage renal disease in the United States. Am J Kidney Dis. 2012;59(1 Suppl 1):A7, e1-420.
2. Smith JM, Martz K, Blydt-Hansen TD. Pediatric kidney transplant practice patterns and outcome benchmarks, 1987-2010: a report of the North American Pediatric Renal Trials and Collaborative Studies. Pediatr Transplant. 2013; 17(2):149-57.
3. Churchill BM, Jayanthi RV, McLorie GA, et al. Pediatric renal transplantation into the abnormal urinary tract. Pediatr Nephrol. 1996;10(1):113-20.
4. Gjertson DW, Cecka JM. Determinants of long-term survival of pediatric kidney grafts reported to the United Network for Organ Sharing kidney transplant registry. Pediatr Transplant. 2001;5(1):5-15.
5. Ellis EN, Martz K, Talley L, et al. Factors related to long-term renal transplant function in children. Pediatr Nephrol. 2008;23(7):1149-55.
6. Salvatierra O, Jr, Millan M, Concepcion W. Pediatric renal transplantation with considerations for successful outcomes. Seminars in pediatric surgery. 2006; 15(3):208-17.
7. Gulleroglu K, Baskin E, Bayrakci US, et al. Antibody-mediated rejection and treatment in pediatric patients: one center's experience. Exp Clin Transplant. 2013;11(5):404-7.
8. Twombley K, Thach L, Ribeiro A, et al. Acute antibody-mediated rejection in pediatric kidney transplants: a single center experience. Pediatr Transplant. 2013;17(7):E149-55.
9. Hsu DT. Biological and psychological differences in the child and adolescent transplant recipient. Pediatr Transplant. 2005;9(3):416-21.
10. Grenda R, Watson A, Trompeter R, et al. A randomized trial to assess the impact of early steroid withdrawal on growth in pediatric renal transplantation: the TWIST study. Am J Transplant. 2010;10(4):828-36.
11. Hocker B, Tonshoff B. Calcineurin inhibitor-free immunosuppression in pediatric renal transplantation: a viable option? Paediatr Drugs. 2011;13(1):49-69.
12. Ganschow R, Pape L, Sturm E, et al. Growing experience with mTOR inhibitors in pediatric solid organ transplantation. Pediatr Transplant. 2013;17(7):694-706.
13. Sarwal MM, Cecka JM, Millan MT, et al. Adult-size kidneys without acute tubular necrosis provide exceedingly superior long-term graft outcomes for infants and small children: a single center and UNOS analysis. United Network for Organ Sharing. Transplantation. 2000;70(12):1728-36.

14. Van Arendonk KJ, James NT, Locke JE, et al. Late graft loss among pediatric recipients of DCD kidneys. Clin J Am Soc Nephrol. 2011;6(11):2705-11.
15. Sureshkumar KK, Reddy CS, Nghiem DD, et al. Superiority of pediatric en bloc renal allografts over living donor kidneys: a long-term functional study. Transplantation. 2006;82(3):348-53.
16. Lau KK, Berg GM, Schjoneman YG, et al. Pediatric en bloc kidney transplantation into pediatric recipients. Pediatr Transplant. 2010;14(1):100-104.
17. Butani L, Troppmann C, Perez RV. Outcomes of children receiving en bloc renal transplants from small pediatric donors. Pediatr Transplant. 2013;17(1):55-8.
18. Tejani A, Sullivan EK, Alexander S, et al. Posttransplant deaths and factors that influence the mortality rate in North American children. Transplantation. 1994;57(4):547-53.
19. US Renal Data System, USRDS 2013 Annual Data Report: Atlas of Chronic Kidney Disease and End-Stage Renal Disease in the United States, National Institutes of Health, National Institute of Diabetes and Digestive and Kidney Diseases, Bethesda, MD, 2013.
20. Dharnidharka VR, Stablein DM, Harmon WE. Post-transplant infections now exceed acute rejection as cause for hospitalization: a report of the NAPRTCS. Am J Transplant. 2004;4(3):384-9.
21. Puliyanda DP, Stablein DM, Dharnidharka VR. Younger age and antibody induction increase the risk for infection in pediatric renal transplantation: a NAPRTCS report. Am J Transplant. 2007;7(3):662-6.
22. Dharnidharka VR, Agodoa LY, Abbott KC. Risk factors for hospitalization for bacterial or viral infection in renal transplant recipients–an analysis of USRDS data. Am J Transplant. 2007;7(3):653-61.
23. Parekh RS, Carroll CE, Wolfe RA, et al. Cardiovascular mortality in children and young adults with end-stage kidney disease. J Pediatr. 2002;141(2):191-7.
24. Silverstein DM, Palmer J, Polinsky MS, et al. Risk factors for hyperlipidemia in long-term pediatric renal transplant recipients. Pediatr Nephrol. 2000;14(2):105-10.
25. Mynarek M, Hussein K, Kreipe HH, et al. Malignancies after pediatric kidney transplantation: more than PTLD? Pediatr Nephrol. 2013. [Epub a head of print].
26. Opelz G, Dohler B. Lymphomas after solid organ transplantation: a collaborative transplant study report. Am J Transplant. 2004;4(2):222-30.
27. Engels EA, Pfeiffer RM, Fraumeni JF, Jr, et al. Spectrum of cancer risk among US solid organ transplant recipients. JAMA. 2011;306(17):1891-901.
28. Reshef R, Vardhanabhuti S, Luskin MR, et al. Reduction of immunosuppression as initial therapy for posttransplantation lymphoproliferative disorder (bigstar). Am J Transplant. 2011;11(2):336-47.
29. Gross TG, Orjuela MA, Perkins SL, et al. Low-dose chemotherapy and rituximab for posttransplant lymphoproliferative disease (PTLD): a Children's Oncology Group Report. Am J Transplant. 2012;12(11):3069-75.
30. Fine RN, Martz K, Stablein D. What have 20 years of data from the North American Pediatric Renal Transplant Cooperative Study taught us about growth following renal transplantation in infants, children, and adolescents with end-stage renal disease? Pediatr Nephrol. 2010;25(4):739-46.
31. Boucek MM, Edwards LB, Keck BM, et al. The Registry of the International Society for Heart and Lung Transplantation: Sixth Official Pediatric Report – 2003. J Heart Lung Transplant. 2003;22(6):636-52.

32. Bartosh SM, Leverson G, Robillard D, et al. Long-term outcomes in pediatric renal transplant recipients who survive into adulthood. Transplantation. 2003;76(8):1195-200.
33. Van Arendonk KJ, James NT, Orandi BJ, et al. Order of donor type in pediatric kidney transplant recipients requiring retransplantation. Transplantation. 2013;96(5):487-93.

CHAPTER

6

Considerations for the Management of Older Kidney Transplant Recipients

Meredith J Aull, Sandip Kapur

ABSTRACT

Older kidney transplant candidates and recipients represent a complex and challenging patient population who have the potential to benefit greatly from kidney transplantation. Despite the cautious immunosuppression regimens utilized historically for older kidney transplant recipients, induction therapy plays an important role in the management of this population, particularly because of the increasing utilization of marginal donor organs. Living donor kidney transplantation affords older patients the best outcomes; however, for those without that option, appropriate matching of older transplant candidates with marginal organs in order to reduce time on the waiting list and on dialysis appears to be the best option to reduce mortality while waiting for a transplant. There is still much to be learned about the selection of older patients for transplant and the peri- and postoperative management of those patients selected to qualify for transplantation.

INTRODUCTION

As of the 2009, 48% of the incident end-stage renal disease (ESRD) population was aged 65 years or older, and 36% of all new patients with ESRD were over the age of 70.[1] Despite these large numbers, only 3.4% of patients aged 70–79 and 0.5% of those aged 80 or older had been added to the kidney transplant waiting list. It is well-established that kidney transplantation for older patients (age $\geq$65) with ESRD significantly reduces mortality when compared to remaining on dialysis and on the waiting list.[2,3] Accordingly, the percentage of both living donor (LD) and deceased donor (DD) kidneys allocated to patients age 65 and older have more than doubled over a period of 10 years.[4] Numerous studies have confirmed that renal transplant in this older population is safe and graft outcomes are similar to those observed in younger populations up to 5 years post-transplant.[5,6] However, the remodeling of the immune system with aging, known as immunosenescence, presents a potential challenge when determining an immunosuppression regimen for these patients, and no optimal protocol for older patients has been identified.[7] The choice of an induction agent in the older population remains unclear; no prospective, randomized induction trials have been performed in this population, therefore we must rely on single center reports and analysis of registry data for insight into the best options.

Increased mortality due to infection has been documented in older transplant recipients,[8,9] and increased age is a risk factor for malignancy in the post-transplant period.[10,11] Although acute rejection (AR) may be less common in older patients compared to younger patients, the impact of rejection is especially concerning in older transplant recipients. The higher utilization of marginal donor kidneys in the older population [such as expanded criteria donor (ECD) kidneys] must be taken into consideration, as allografts from older donors may be more immunogenic than better quality allografts,[12] and older recipients may face an increased risk of graft loss[12-14] and/or mortality[13,14] after AR.

There is much still to be learned about the management of older kidney transplant recipients. Interested readers are encouraged to examine the proceedings of a workshop published in October 2012,[15] which nicely summarizes the many questions that surround transplantation of older adults.

CONSIDERATIONS FOR SELECTION OF OLDER KIDNEY TRANSPLANT CANDIDATES

As would be expected in an aging population, older kidney transplant candidates have a high degree of comorbid conditions such as diabetes mellitus, hypertension, hypercholesterolemia, and cardiovascular disease. Often, the older patient's transplant candidacy depends on the severity of these comorbidities and their associated complications. Approximately half of kidney transplant candidates over the age of 60 on the waiting list will die before receiving a transplant.[16] Interpretation of published outcomes after transplantation in older patients is difficult due to potential selection bias in the patients accepted for transplantation.

Grams and colleagues found that access to transplantation is particularly poor in the older population (≥65 years) and that a risk-prediction model could help to identify suitable candidates in combination with appropriate referral.[17] Little data are available on the criteria used to either accept or deny older kidney transplant candidates for addition to the waiting list. Lenihan and colleagues analyzed 123 patients aged 65 years or older to identify factors associated with wait-listing.[18] Factors associated with denial of listing included older age (OR 1.29 per year over 65), coronary artery disease (OR 8.57), and poor mobility (OR 13.97).

In addition to the comorbidities in this population, additional challenges that may impact the older transplant population include frailty, falls, and functional and/or cognitive impairment. A recent area of interest is the quantification of frailty using the criteria developed by Fried,[19] which measures frailty using five components: exhaustion, weight loss, low activity, slow walk, and grip strength. Johansen and colleagues studied 2,275 dialysis patients who participated in the Dialysis Morbidity and Mortality Wave 2 Study,[20] and found that two-thirds of the patients met the criteria for frailty (utilizing the modification of the original Fried's criteria by Woods).[21] Risk factors for frailty included older age, female gender, and being on hemodialysis (as opposed to peritoneal dialysis). Frail dialysis patients were at higher risk for death (HR 2.24, CI 1.60–3.15) and for a combined outcome of death or hospitalization (HR 1.63, CI 1.41–1.87). Dialysis patients with better physical function also have lower post-transplant hospitalization and mortality.[22]

Garonzik-Wang and colleagues prospectively identified 25% of 183 patients selected to undergo kidney transplantation as meeting the criteria for frailty (defined as meeting 3 or more of the criteria, including shrinking, exhaustion, low physical activity, slowed walking speed, and weakness).[23] In this study, frailty was shown to be an independent risk factor for post-transplant delayed graft function. Importantly, frailty may help to identify risk of poorer post-transplant outcomes, regardless of patient age.

Risk Stratification

There are several tools available that may assist with risk stratification for kidney transplant candidates or recipients. The Charlson Comorbidity Index (CCI) is a tool that may serve as a surrogate marker of comorbidities in the older population. CCI is a validated method to stratify comorbid conditions that affect the risk for mortality in various patient populations, which has been successfully applied to predict outcomes in living donor and standard criteria donor (SCD) kidney transplant recipients.[24,25]

A recent risk stratification tool was studied by Gill and colleagues in 25,468 patients with ESRD to assess cardiovascular risk in those aged 65 years and older.[26] All patients with diabetes were considered high risk, and patients without diabetes were categorized based on presence/history of ischemic heart disease, congestive heart failure, cerebrovascular accident, or peripheral vascular disease, receiving 1 point for each condition. Patients with zero points were considered low risk, with one point were intermediate risk, and with two or more points were considered high risk. Over the course of a median of 2.7 years, 43% of patients received a transplant, 25% died on the waiting list, and 6% were removed from the waiting list. One-third of patients died after transplant (27% of low risk, 34% of intermediate risk, and 41% of high risk patients), and among all risk groups, the risk of death was highest in recipients of ECD kidneys, followed by SCD and living donor kidneys. In this study, delayed graft function was an independent risk factor for death after transplantation.

Survival data are also often difficult to interpret for older kidney transplant recipients due to the general increased risk of death with aging. In order to address this issue, Foucher and colleagues compared mortality rates of kidney transplant recipients to rates in the general population in order to assess for excess mortality that could be attributed to transplantation.[27] Interestingly, recipient age was not responsible for the excess mortality observed in kidney transplant recipients. Instead, risk factors for mortality included pretransplant DM, detectable historical peak panel reactive antibodies, organ donor death from a cerebrovascular accident, and delayed graft function. Karim and colleagues studied 19,103 kidney transplants performed in the United Kingdom between 2001 and 2012, who had a median follow-up of 4.4 years after transplant.[28] As one might expect, the investigators found an increasing mortality rate with every decade of aging (5.8% in those <50 years, 14.2% for those 50–59, 22.0% for those 60–69, 31.9% for those 70–79, and 45.5% for those 80 years and over). The most common causes of death in kidney recipients over the age of 70 were cardiac (21.2%), infection (21.2%), and malignancy (20.2%). Living donor transplantation afforded patients over 70 years a survival benefit, while risk factors for mortality included history of cerebrovascular accident, myocardial infarction, cancer, peripheral vascular disease, and congestive cardiac failure (which was the most significant prognosticator of mortality).

Faravardeh and colleagues assessed patient and graft outcome in 364 kidney transplant recipients aged 65 years or older, comparing them to 2 younger cohorts [(age <50 (n = 2900) and aged 50–64 (n = 1218))].[29] Risk factors for mortality in a subset of patients transplanted after 2000, who received induction with rATG, and calcineurin inhibitor and mycophenolate maintenance therapy (steroid-free) included coronary artery disease, allograft failure, and peripheral vascular disease. Risk factors for graft loss included congestive heart failure and AR >1 year after transplant.

Analysis of 160 patients over the age of 70 years who received a kidney transplant between 2000 and 2005 analyzed variables that might predict outcome in this group of patients.[30] The median CCI score in this population was 3.0, and was not associated with patient survival. The majority of patients received a triple-drug immunosuppression regimen with CsA, mycophenolate mofetil (MMF), and steroids, and only 24% received IL2RA induction therapy. AR occurred in 22% of patients within the first 90 days; however, this did not influence patient or graft survival. Risk factors for post-transplant mortality included age at time of transplant [hazard ratio (HR) 1.09/year], time on dialysis (HR 1.29/year), and diagnosis of diabetes at the time of transplant (HR 1.78). The development of an abnormal oral glucose tolerance test at 10-week post-transplant (which was abnormal in 39.6% of those tested who were not previously diagnosed with DM) was also associated with reduced post-transplant survival. The median survival for this population was 7.9 years after transplant. The 5-year survival for older transplant recipients reported in the 2009 OPTN/SRTR annual report was 77.6% for recipients of LD allografts and 65.1% for recipients of DD allografts.[4]

CONSIDERATIONS FOR LIVING VS DECEASED DONOR TRANSPLANTATION IN THE OLDER POPULATION

It has been increasingly common to perform living donor kidney transplants in older patients, and this has also led to an increase in the number of older living kidney donors as well. In the study of Gill and colleagues mentioned above, receipt of a living donor kidney transplant provided an immediate lower risk of death as compared to remaining on dialysis for patients at low or intermediate cardiac risk.[26] For high-risk patients, the number of days to equal survival was 130 days when receiving a living donor allograft, 368 days with a SCD transplant, and 521 days if receiving an ECD transplant, demonstrating the benefit of living donor kidney transplantation in this high-risk patient population. Regardless of donor source, however, patients receiving a transplant had a reduced long-term risk of mortality as compared to remaining on dialysis.

Jassal and colleagues utilized a decision analysis model to evaluate the costs and benefits of kidney transplant vs dialysis for older patients (defined as aged 65 years and over).[31] As would be expected, patients derived greater benefit from early transplantation as opposed to a prolonged wait on dialysis. From a cost perspective, deceased donor transplant was more attractive for patients aged 65 years and older if they were at a transplant center where the waiting time was 2 years or less, while for living donor kidney transplantation, transplantation was beneficial up to age 80.

An interesting model of deceased donor kidney transplantation is the Eurotransplant Senior Program (ESP), which was established in Europe to increase utilization of older donor kidneys and reduce waiting times for older candidates. The program is referred to as the "Old to Old" program, since it is designed for transplant candidates aged 65 and older to receive a kidney transplant from a deceased donor aged 65 and older.[32] Implemented in January of 1999, the allocation scheme was designed to match the metabolic demand of the transplant recipient with the excretory capacity of the donor organ. The program is limited to first transplant recipients who are unsensitized [defined as panel reactive antibody (PRA) <5%]. If the donor's creatinine clearance was <70 mL/min, both kidneys are transplanted into one recipient. Results of the first year of ESP found that the program reduced waiting time of patients over 65 from 943 days in 1998 to 707 days in 1999, while waiting times remained stable for patients younger than 65. Cold ischemia time was significantly shorter in the ESP group

(12 vs 19 h; $P = 0.03$). Delayed graft function, primary nonfunction, and AR rates were similar between ESP participants and controls, as was patient and graft survival.

More recently, the effectiveness of the ESP was evaluated by Frei and colleagues,[33] who compared outcomes between 3 groups (ESP group, any-to-old group, where a 60–64 year old candidate received any age donor, and the old-to-any group, where a kidney from a donor aged 65 or above went to a recipient of any age). The ESP group had a shorter waiting time for their transplant compared to the "any-to-old" group (3.6 vs 4.6 years; $P<0.001$), received more depleting induction therapy (20.8% vs 12.2% vs 12.9%, respectively), had a lower cold ischemia time (11.9 vs >17 h in both other groups; $P<0.05$), and had a significantly higher rate of rejection as compared to the "any-to-old" group (29.1% vs 20.1%; $P<0.001$). Patients in the ESP group also had a lower rate of delayed graft function compared to the old-to-any group (29.7 vs 36.2%; $P = 0.047$). The ESP group had the lowest 1 and 5-year patient survival rates with 86% and 60% compared to 88% and 71% for "old-to-any" ($P = 0.049$) and 90% and 74% for "any-to-old" ($P<0.001$). Death-censored graft survival in ESP was not different from "old-to-any" (1 year: 83% vs 81% and 5 year: 67% for both; $P = 0.552$), but significantly different from "any-to-old" (1 year 90% and 5 year 81%; $P<0.001$), as would be expected based on quality of younger donor kidneys.

Rao and colleagues analyzed 5,667 elderly kidney transplant candidates (defined as ages 70 years and older) who were wait-listed between 1990 and 2004. By the end of 2005, 2,078 (36.7%) had received a deceased donor transplant, while only 360 (6.4%) had received a living donor transplant.[3] As compared to the patients that remained on the waiting list, transplanted patients had a 41% overall lower risk of death (RR = 0.59, CI 0.53–0.65; $P<0.0001$). Those patients that received expanded donor organs also had a significantly lower risk of mortality (RR = 0.75; $P<0.0001$). The time to an equal risk of death between transplanted patients vs staying on the waiting list was 125 days, while the time to equal survival was just under 2 years (1.8 years). Elderly patients with diabetes or hypertension as their cause of ESRD also experienced great benefit from transplantation.

Schold and Meier-Kriesche attempted to answer the question of whether patients should be willing to accepted expanded donor organs in order to be transplanted more quickly.[34] They found that older patients (65 years of age and older) have a better life expectancy by accepting an ECD organ within 2 years of the onset of their ESRD, as compared to being on dialysis for 4 years and receiving either a standard criteria organ or even a living donor organ, because the benefit of waiting for a better organ was negated by the additional time on dialysis. In addition, this analysis found that patients with diabetes should be transplanted as early as possible, to avoid effects of dialysis.

Older Living Donors

An analysis of 80,347 kidney donors who donated in the United States between April 1, 1994 and March 31, 2009 found that only 3.8% of living donors were ages 60 years or older.[35] Donors were followed for a median of 6.3 years, and were matched to National Health and Nutrition Examination Survey (NHANES) III participants. The authors found no evidence that donors over the age of 50 years are at higher risk of surgical mortality associated with donation, and donors had similar survival to the matched cohort.

Several centers, including our own, have analyzed kidney donor and recipient outcomes associated with acceptance of older living kidney donors (age cutoff varies by study). Our center's experience found that utilization of older living donors (aged 50 years and older, n = 143) led to equivalent patient and graft survival compared to outcomes in recipients of younger donor organs (n = 319), while graft function (as defined by eGFR) was lower in the recipients of older donor organs at 5 years post-transplant.[36] The older donors themselves, up to 3 years after donation, showed no progressive decline in renal function.

Berger and colleagues studied outcomes when 219 donors age 70 and older served as living donors.[37] Mean recipient age of the older donor kidneys was 56 years. When compared to a matched cohort that received a kidney from a living donor aged 50–59 years, the graft failure rate was higher in those receiving a kidney from a donor ≥70 years, however, when the analysis was limited to recipients over the age of 65, no difference was observed. When the recipients of the older kidneys were compared to a matched group of recipients of non-ECD deceased donor organs aged 50–59, graft survival was similar between the groups. The outcomes of the over 70 kidney donors were compared to matched controls obtained from the NHANES III cohort, and the kidney donors were found to have better patient survival.

In a quality of life study of older living kidney donors (defined as 60 years of age or older), findings supported relatively fast recovery of older living donors.[38] At 1 month post-donation, older patients scored better than younger patients in the domains of "bodily pain," "role physical," and "vitality."

ACUTE REJECTION

The deterioration of the immune system with aging, known as immunosenescence is an important factor to consider when designing an immunosuppression regimen. However, it is also very important to recognize that the older deceased donor organs often received by older transplant candidates have increased immunogenicity and a reduced ability to recover from damage. Interested readers are referred to an excellent review of immunosenescence by Heinbokel and colleagues.[39] Several studies have shown that the impact of AR episodes on patient and graft survival is more pronounced in older kidney transplant recipients.[12,14] Heldal and colleagues categorized first kidney transplants performed at their center between 1990 and 2005 into three groups, elderly (defined as ≥70 years of age; $n = 354$), senior (age 60–69 years; $n = 577$), and control (age 45–54 years; $n = 563$), and analyzed risk factors for graft loss and death.[12] Median patient survival was 5.3 years in the elderly, 8.0 years in the seniors, and 17.1 years in the control group. AR within the first 3 months of transplant was a strong predictor of death in both the elderly and senior groups, and the leading cause of death in the elderly group in the first 3 months was infection. Interestingly, of the 11 patients who died of infection within those first 3 months, 8 had previously been treated for AR.

Although based on an older immunosuppression regimen (cyclosporine, prednisone, ± azathioprine, no induction), de Fijter and colleagues also observed increased immunogenicity of older donor kidneys, leading to a negative impact on graft survival.[14] The authors proposed that older donor kidneys have an impaired ability to recover after rejection.

Choice of Immunosuppression Regimen

Finding a balance between prevention of AR and over-immunosuppression in older renal transplant recipients remains an important challenge. The choice to utilize induction therapy in older kidney transplant recipients, as well as choice of induction agent remains a controversial topic in this patient population, which may in part be due to poor representation of older subjects in clinical trials. Blosser and colleagues studied kidney transplant clinical trials to assess the relationship of patient age and the trials' exclusion criteria.[40] The study found that of 573 trials (representing 87,222 participants), 30% had exclusion criteria related to age, and 16% specifically excluded patients over the age of 65. Immunosuppression trials were more likely to exclude the elderly (OR 2.40), as were those published in high impact journals (OR 1.74).

Heldal and Midtvedt recommend a strategy based on the combination of donor and recipient risk factors,[41] similar to the study by Gill and colleagues described below.[42] Choice of regimen is challenging since although increasing recipient age decreases the frequency of rejection, increasing donor age increases the frequency,[43] therefore making for a challenging balance.

The European Senior Transplant Program studied age-dependent immune response by comparing 26 patients aged 65 or older receiving a kidney transplant from a donor aged 65 or older to 74 patients younger than 65 who received a transplant from a donor younger than 65.[44] Before transplant, the older patients had elevated numbers of natural killer, memory T, and activated cytotoxic T cells, and significantly reduced numbers of B, naïve T, and helper T cells. Older patients had an initially pronounced immune response when given an older donor kidney, with increased memory T, activated cytotoxic T, and alloreactive T cells, and T-cell alloreactivity was more pronounced in the elderly patients throughout follow-up. This serves to demonstrate that older organs may increase the older patient's immune response to transplantation, with resultant need for enhanced immunosuppression as described below.

Induction Therapy

Between 2003 and 2008, 14,820 kidney transplant recipients aged 60 or older in the United States received induction therapy with rabbit antithymocyte globulin (rATG) (48.2%), interleukin 2 receptor antibodies (IL2RA) (41.9%), or alemtuzumab (9.9%).[42] Over that 5-year time period, approximately 25% of patients over 60 years of age were off of steroids at the time of discharge, although these rates were higher in patients receiving lymphocyte-depleting therapy (rATG or alemtuzumab). Over 75% of this older patient population transplanted in 2008 received some form of induction therapy.[42] The use of alemtuzumab for induction therapy in older patients (>60 years of age) has been associated with higher rates of AR, graft loss, and mortality after kidney transplantation.[42,45]

Recent analysis of the United States Renal Data System database looked at use of induction therapy in kidney transplant recipients age 65 and older, and may be helpful in guiding choice of induction agent in the older population.[46] The analysis showed statistically higher AR rate at 1 year in basiliximab and alemtuzumab treated patients (6.8% each vs 5.1% with daclizumab, 5.0% with rATG), although the percentage of patients with AR is lower than that typically seen in younger recipients. The percent of patients who were steroid-free at discharge was variable (14.9% basiliximab, 11.6% daclizumab, 36.2% rATG, 72% alemtuzumab).[46] The study from Gill and colleagues also reported increased rates of AR with IL2RA induction (1 year 7.3% with rATG vs 10.5% with IL2RA).[42] In addition, their study also showed an increased risk of death and worse long-term graft survival in patients receiving IL2RA induction. This effect was not seen after correction for AR, suggesting that the avoidance of AR could carry significant advantage for long-term patient and graft outcomes in older kidney recipients. Other groups have also reported the negative effects of AR on outcomes in older allograft recipients.[12,14] Therefore, although rejection rates tend to be lower in older recipients, the effect of rejection can be devastating to this patient population. It is important to recognize that older patients receiving no induction therapy and cyclosporine-based maintenance regimens may experience up to a 50% rate of AR.[47]

In an analysis of patients aged 60 and older who received a DD kidney transplant from 2003 to 2008, Gill and colleagues stratified the transplants by risk of both the recipient and donor.[42] Recipients were considered high immunologic risk if they had a peak PRA above 20%, while donors were considered high risk if they met criteria as being an ECD or DCD donor, or if the cold ischemia time was >24 h. In this analysis, it was shown that both high-risk recipient/high-risk donor and low-risk recipient/high-risk donor combinations benefit from rATG induction in terms of freedom from rejection, while the low-risk recipient/high-risk donor group had a trend toward an increased risk of death if they received IL2RA induction. In this analysis, the majority of patients were discharged from their initial transplant admission on tacrolimus, MMF, and steroids.

Khanmoradi and colleagues retrospectively analyzed 137 patients ≥65 years of age (elderly group) at time of a deceased donor kidney transplant to 276 patients under the age of 65 (non-elderly group).[48] All patients received rATG induction therapy in combination with a calcineurin inhibitor (tacrolimus or cyclosporine), mycophenolate mofetil/mycophenolate sodium and corticosteroids. The elderly group (mean age 70.8 years) received a total weight-based rATG dose of 5.3 mg/kg compared to 5.6 mg/kg in the nonelderly group (mean age 52.5 years) ($P = 0.04$). There was no significant difference in rates of cytomegalovirus infection, urinary tract infection, pneumonia, or surgical wound complications between groups. Malignancy occurred in 5.1% of elderly patients vs 2.2% of nonelderly patients (P = NS). Biopsy proven AR occurred in 13.1% of elderly patients at 1-year vs 16.7% of non-elderly patients (P = NS). Three-year death censored graft survival was similar between groups; however, 3-year patient survival was inferior in the elderly group ($P = 0.002$).

Heldal and colleagues studied 232 patients who received a kidney transplant from a donor who was aged 60 years or older.[49] All patients received triple therapy with a calcineurin inhibitor, MMF, and steroids, and either had or had not received IL2RA induction therapy. Mean age of the recipient cohort was 64.6 years, with a median follow-up of 4.4 years after transplant. Patients who received no induction had an increase in early AR (within 90 days) [41% vs 20% in those receiving induction; Odds Ratio (OR) 2.42] as well as steroid-resistant rejection (22% vs 3%; OR 8.04). Patients receiving induction had superior 2-year uncensored (87% vs 70%; $P = 0.001$) and death-censored (95% vs 79%; $P<0.001$) graft survival.

Maintenance Therapy

As mentioned earlier, no ideal immunosuppression regimen has been defined for older kidney transplant recipients, and much controversy exists as to the ideal way to manage this patient population. Regardless of the regimen chosen, it may be more important to recognize the issues that can affect drug disposition in these patients, including age-related alterations in cytochrome P450 and P-glycoprotein expression/activity, decreased liver mass, changes in body composition, increased risk of polypharmacy due to comorbid conditions (leading to drug interactions or overlapping toxicities), suboptimal post-transplant kidney function, and increased susceptibility to adverse effects.[50] All of these require careful monitoring and adjustment of the medication regimen on a routine basis.

One study of calcineurin inhibitor exposure in kidney transplant recipients of varying age groups found that as compared to young (aged 18–34) and middle-aged (35–64) patients, older aged patients (65–84) had higher normalized tacrolimus and cyclosporine troughs (17% higher than middle-aged, 58–68% higher than young patients) despite receiving lower doses of the drugs (1–2 mg/day less tacrolimus; 100 mg/day less cyclosporine).[51]

Alterations in calcineurin inhibitor metabolism and distribution in older transplant recipients are most concerning due to the potential for neurologic effects such as headache, tremors, sleep disturbance, confusion, and lethargy, which tend to be worse in tacrolimus-treated patients. In severe cases, patients may experience psychoses, hallucinations, blindness, seizures, cerebellar ataxia, motor weakness, and leukoencephalopathy.[52] It is important to recognize that the neurologic complications may not correlate with trough concentrations in the older population. Posterior reversible encephalopathy syndrome (PRES) is the characteristic imaging presentation seen in patients with calcineurin inhibitor-induced neurotoxicity. Besenski and colleagues reviewed their center's kidney transplant population to assess those that requiring magnetic resonance imaging for CNS symptoms and found that 10.3% of the population required imaging in the post-transplant setting.[53] Indications for imaging included altered mental status in 38%, headache in 27%, infection in 16%, and seizures in 12%. The most common acute findings on MR included acute infarcts (12%) and infection (6.5%), while the majority of other cases had more chronic changes.

Although older patients were not specifically excluded from large multi-center trials of corticosteroid withdrawal (CSWD), this patient population appears to represent < 5% of patients in these trials.[54-56] However, some of this population could potentially benefit from CSWD given the high prevalence of comorbidities in these patients that might be exacerbated by steroid use, such as bone loss, glucose intolerance or diabetes.[15]

COMPLICATIONS OF TRANSPLANTATION IN THE OLDER POPULATION

New Onset Diabetes Mellitus

New onset diabetes mellitus (NODM) is an important complication for organ transplant recipients. Although the terminology and definition of NODM varies in the transplant literature, it is an important risk factor for post-transplant morbidity and mortality regardless of the exact definition used. Increasing age is one of the most important nonmodifiable risk factors for NODM,[57–59] and thus the older kidney transplant population is at high risk of developing this complication, adding to the complex management of such patients. Addressing modifiable risk factors such as obesity and choice of immunosuppression regimen may be helpful to either reduce risk and/or manage the complication once it occurs.[60,61]

Infections

As a transplant community, we recognize that treatment of AR predisposes patients to infectious complications, leading us to reintroduce opportunistic infection prophylaxis. On the other hand, we also see AR precipitated by infection (i.e. in the setting of reduced immunosuppression in patients with polyomavirus-associated nephropathy). Consideration of infectious complications post-transplant is of great importance, as it has been shown that older renal transplant recipients may be significantly more susceptible to bacterial infections,[62] and the risk for infectious death increases dramatically in older transplant recipients.[9] USRDS data on patients wait-listed or transplanted between 1988 and 1997 showed that compared to the patients remaining on the waiting list, transplant patients had an increased risk of death from infectious causes.[9] However, it is important to note that these patients would have received older immunosuppression regimens with likely higher rejection rates and resultant treatment, which may have influenced the outcome, and thus may not be representative of experience under modern immunosuppression regimens.

Dharnidharka and colleagues assessed infection within the first post-transplant year in 64,751 kidney recipients transplanted between 1991 and 1998 by using Medicare claims.[63] Older adults (defined as those age 51 years and older) had the highest risk of infection, and there was a higher adjusted risk of bacterial infection in the elderly (specifically septicemia and cellulitis).

A study about the causes of death-censored graft failure performed by Parasuraman and colleagues correlated an increase in infection-related causes of graft loss with the increased utilization of induction therapy over the period of 1990 to 2006. The risk of infection-related graft loss was highest in patients 65 and older, and this was the only age group where the risk of graft loss from infection exceeded the risk from rejection.[64] Multivariable analysis of the risk factors for infection-related graft loss included urologic complications (OR 8.77), polyomavirus infection (OR 2.55), AR (OR 1.85), induction therapy (OR 1.66), treatment for rejection (OR 1.25), and age (OR 1.02). It is important to recognize that both acute kidney injury and medication-induced nephrotoxicity may contribute to graft loss in the setting of serious infection.

Malignancy

As seen in the general population, increasing age is a risk factor for the development of malignancy after transplantation. Farrugia and colleagues analyzed malignancy-related mortality in 19,103 kidney transplants performed in the United Kingdom between 2001 and 2012, who had a median of 4.4 years of follow-up.[65] Overall, 10.9% of patients died over the follow-up period, and 18% of those deaths were due to malignancy. Independent risk factors for malignancy-related death included increasing age, pretransplant history of malignancy, and having received a deceased donor kidney transplant. The breakdown of malignancy-related death by age revealed the following: age <50 years, 0.8%; aged 50–59, 2.5%; aged 60–69, 4.8%; aged 70–79, 6.5%; aged 80 or older, 9.1%.

Clarke and colleagues studies lymphoma subtypes developing in transplant recipients between 1987 and 2008.[66] For all organ transplant types, recipients aged 65 years and above had increased risk of the following B-cell lymphoma subtypes: Burkitt's lymphoma/leukemia [standardized incidence ratio (SIR) 8.1], diffuse large B-cell lymphoma (SIR 5.8), lymphoplasmacytic lymphoma (SIR 3.5) and marginal zone (SIR 2.5). Increased risk of T-cell lymphoma subtypes included primary cutaneous anaplastic large cell lymphoma (SIR 17.5), all T-cell lymphoma (SIR 3.2), non-Hodgkin's lymphoma (NHL), not otherwise specified (SIR 4.4) and all NHL (2.8). Other investigators have observed a relationship between older age at transplant and the risk of myeloma and leukemia.[67]

Readmission

Another important consideration for transplantation of older adults is risk of readmission after transplantation. Patients over the age of 65 have been shown to have a higher rate of readmission in the year after transplant (31.8% vs 10.9% in patients <65; P<0.001).[68] Frailty has also been shown to be an important predictor of post-transplant readmission.[69] Analysis of 383 kidney recipients at Johns Hopkins found that 18.8% were frail at the time of transplant, and the rate of early hospital readmission (within 30 days of initial discharge) was significantly higher in the frail (45.8% vs 28.0% in nonfrail; P = 0.005). Frailty independently predicted a 61% higher risk of early readmission.[69]

Grams and colleagues studied the reasons for rehospitalization in patients aged 65 or older at time of transplant[70] by analyzing 27,247 Medicare primary kidney transplant recipients. The top 5 reasons included kidney/ureter/pelvis/bladder/procedures, infection, circulatory disorders, rehabilitation, and miscellaneous reasons. Only the reason of rehabilitation was unique to the older population. The authors also looked at the number of excess inpatient days within the first year of transplant, and defined poor outcome are >120 excess inpatient days or death. Risk factors for poor outcome in the older population included age, time on dialysis, time hospitalized within the year prior to transplant, diabetes or hypertension as cause of ESRD, and congestive heart failure.

QUALITY OF LIFE

Quality of life studies in older kidney transplant recipients have conflicting results, likely due to differences in patients characteristics such as type of transplant (i.e. living vs deceased) and comorbidities. Cornella and colleagues studied 52 kidney transplant recipients over the age of 60 using the SF-36 form, and compared the responses to national age and gender norms (Italy).[71] Although not clearly indicated, it appears all transplant recipients were at least 1 year post-transplant at the time of survey administration. The case mix breakdown of the surveyed transplant patients included 1 standard, 7 mild, 24 moderate, and 20 severe; although this categorization is not well described, it can be inferred that the majority of these patients had significant comorbidities. Compared to the national controls, both female and male transplant recipients had lower scores in the areas of social activity and general health perception, and increased perception of pain, while male respondents also had lower psychophysical energy.

Humar and colleagues administered the SF-36 at 1-year post-transplant to 149 patients under the age of 65 and 42 patients age 65 and older.[72] Over 40% of patients in each group had received their transplant from a living donor. Compared to national norms, the combined groups of transplant recipients scored higher in the areas of general health perception, social functioning, and mental health, and interestingly, the older kidney recipients scored better than the young kidney recipients in the areas of social functioning and mental health. Kniepeiss and colleagues review three studies addressing quality of life in kidney transplantation, and found that using the SF-36, elderly kidney transplant recipients had higher physical function scores as compared to age-adjusted norms.[73]

CONCLUSION

In summary, older kidney transplant candidates and recipients represent a complex and challenging patient population who have the potential to benefit greatly from kidney transplantation. Despite the cautious immunosuppression regimens utilized historically for older kidney transplant recipients, it is clear that induction therapy plays an important role in the management of this population, particularly because of the increasing utilization of marginal donor organs. Living donor kidney transplantation affords older patients the best outcomes; however, for those without that option, appropriate matching of older transplant candidates with marginal organs in order to reduce time on the waiting list and on dialysis appears to be the best option to reduce mortality while waiting for a transplant.

There is still much to be learned about the selection of older patients for transplant and the peri- and postoperative management of those patients selected to qualify for transplantation. Given the strong representation of older patients within the ESRD population, it is of the utmost importance for centers performing such transplants to share what has been learned and well-designed studies are needed to further address areas of uncertainty.

REFERENCES

1. U.S. Renal Data System, USRDS 2011 Annual Data Report: Atlas of Chronic Kidney Disease and End-Stage Renal Disease in the United States, National Institutes of Health, National Institute of Diabetes and Digestive and Kidney Diseases, Bethesda, MD, 2011.
2. Oniscu GC, Brown H, Forsythe JL. How old is old for transplantation? Am J Transplant. 2004;4(12):2067-74.
3. Rao PS, Merion RM, Ashby VB, et al. Renal transplantation in elderly patients older than 70 years of age: results from the Scientific Registry of Transplant Recipients. Transplantation. 2007;83(8):1069-74.
4. 2009 Annual Report for the U.S. Organ Procurement and Transplantation Network and the Scientific Registry of Transplant Recipients: Transplant Data 1999-2008. Department of Health and Human Services, Health Resources and Services Administration, Healthcare Systems Bureau, Division of Transplantation, Rockville, MD; United Network for Organ Sharing, Richmond, VA; University Renal Research and Education Association, Ann Arbor, MI.
5. Sener A, Schweitzer EJ, Munivenkatappa R, et al. Deceased-donor renal transplantation in the geriatric population demonstrates equal graft survival compared with younger recipients. Transplantation. 2009;87(10):1549-54.
6. Mendonça HM, Dos Reis MA, de Castro de Cintra Sesso R, et al. Renal transplantation outcomes: a comparative analysis between elderly and younger recipients. Clin Transplant. 2007;21(6):755-60.
7. Singh N, Nori U, Pesavento T. Kidney transplantation in the elderly. Curr Opin Organ Transplant. 2009;14(4):380-85.
8. Meier-Kriesche HU, Ojo A, Hanson J, et al. Increased immunosuppressive vulnerability in elderly renal transplant recipients. Transplantation. 2000;69(5): 885-9.
9. Meier-Kriesche HU, Ojo AO, Hanson JA, et al. Exponentially increased risk of infectious death in older renal transplant recipients. Kidney Int. 2001;59(4): 1539-43.
10. Kasiske BL, Snyder JJ, Gilbertson DT, et al. Cancer after kidney transplantation in the United States. Am J Transplant. 2004;4(6):905-913.
11. Danpanich E, Kasiske BL. Risk factors for cancer in renal transplant recipients. Transplantation. 1999;68(12):1859-64.
12. de Fijter JW, Mallat MJ, Doxiadis II, et al. Increased immunogenicity and cause of graft loss of old donor kidneys. J Am Soc Nephrol. 2001;12(7):1538-46.
13. Meier-Kriesche H, Ojo AO, Arndorfer JA, et al. Recipient age as an independent risk factor for chronic renal allograft failure. Transplant Proc. 2001;33(1-2):1113-4.

14. Heldal K, Hartmann A, Leivestad T, et al. Clinical outcomes in elderly kidney transplant recipients are related to acute rejection episodes rather than pretransplant comorbidity. Transplantation. 2009;87(7):1045-51.
15. Abecassis M, Bridges ND, Clancy CJ, et al. Solid-organ transplantation in older adults: current status and future research. Am J Transplant. 2012;12(10):2608-22.
16. Schold J, Srinivas TR, Sehgal AR, et al. Half of kidney transplant candidates who are older than 60 years now placed on the waiting list will die before receiving a deceased-donor transplant. Clin J Am Soc Nephrol. 2009;4(7):1239-45.
17. Grams ME, Kucirka LM, Hanrahan CF, et al. Candidacy for kidney transplantation of older adults. J Am Geriatr Soc. 2012;60(1):1-7.
18. Lenihan CR, Hurley MP, Tan JC. Comorbidities and kidney transplant evaluation in the elderly. Am J Nephrol. 2013;38(3):204-11.
19. Fried LP, Tangen CM, Walston J, et al. Frailty in older adults: evidence for a phenotype. J Gerontol A Biol Sci Med Sci. 2001;56(3):M146-56.
20. Johansen KL, Chertow GM, Jin C, et al. Significance of frailty among dialysis patients. J Am Soc Nephrol. 2007;18(11):2960-67.
21. Woods NF, LaCroix AZ, Gray SL, et al. Frailty: emergence and consequences in women aged 65 and older in the Women's Health Initiative Observational Study. J Am Geriatr Soc. 2005;53:1321-30.
22. Kutner NG, Zhang R, Bowles T, et al. Pretransplant physical functioning and kidney patients' risk for posttransplantation hospitalization/death: evidence from a national cohort. Clin J Am Soc Nephrol. 2006;1(4):837-43.
23. Garonzik-Wang JM, Govindan P, Grinnan JW, et al. Frailty and delayed graft function in kidney transplant recipients. Arch Surg. 2012;147(2):190-3.
24. Wu C, Shapiro R, Tan H, Basu A, et al. Kidney transplantation in elderly people: the influence of recipient comorbidity and living kidney donors. J Am Geriatr Soc. 2008;56(2):231-8.
25. Wu C, Evans I, Joseph R, et al. Comorbid conditions in kidney transplantation: association with graft and patient survival. J Am Soc Nephrol. 2005;16(11): 3437-44.
26. Gill JS, Schaeffner E, Chadban S, et al. Quantification of the early risk of death in elderly kidney transplant recipients. Am J Transplant. 2013;13(2):427-32.
27. Foucher Y, Akl A, Rousseau V, et al. An alternative approach to estimate age-related mortality of kidney transplant recipients compared to the general population: results in favor of old-to-old transplantations. Transpl Int. 2014; 27(2):219-25.
28. Karim A, Farrugia D, Cheshire J, et al. Recipient age and risk for mortality after kidney transplantation in England. Transplantation. 2014;97(8):832-8.
29. Faravardeh A, Eickhoff M, Jackson S, et al. Predictors of graft failure and death in elderly kidney transplant recipients. Transplantation. 2013;96(12):1089-96.
30. Heldal K, Hartmann A, Leivestad T, et al. Risk variables associated with the outcome of kidney recipients >70 years of age in the new millennium. Nephrol Dial Transplant. 2011;26(8):2706-11.
31. Jassal SV, Krahn MD, Naglie G, et al. Kidney transplantation in the elderly: a decision analysis. J Am Soc Nephrol. 2003;14(1):187-96.
32. Smits JM, Persijn GG, van Houwelingen HC, et al. Evaluation of the Eurotransplant Senior Program. The results of the first year. Am J Transplant. 2002;2(7):664-70.
33. Frei U, Noeldeke J, Machold-Fabrizii V, et al. Prospective age-matching in elderly kidney transplant recipients - a 5-year analysis of the Eurotransplant Senior Program. Am J Transplant. 2008;8(1):50-57.
34. Schold JD, Meier-Kriesche HU. Which renal transplant candidates should accept marginal kidneys in exchange for a shorter waiting time on dialysis? Clin J Am Soc Nephrol. 2006;1(3):532-8.

35. Segev DL, Muzaale AD, Caffo BS, et al. Perioperative mortality and long-term survival following live kidney donation. JAMA. 2010;303(10):959-66.
36. Balachandran VP, Aull MJ, Charlton M, et al. Kidneys from older living donors provide excellent intermediate-term outcomes after transplantation. Transplantation. 2012;94(5):499-505.
37. Berger JC, Muzaale AD, James N, et al. Living kidney donors ages 70 and older: recipient and donor outcomes. Clin J Am Soc Nephrol. 2011;6(12):2887-93.
38. Klop KW, Dols LF, Weimar W, et al. Quality of life of elderly live kidney donors. Transplantation. 2013;96(7):644-8.
39. Heinbokel T, Elkhal A, Liu G, et al. Immunosenescence and organ transplantation. Transplant Rev (Orlando). 2013;27(3):65-75.
40. Blosser CD, Huverserian A, Bloom RD, et al. Age, exclusion criteria, and generalizability of randomized trials enrolling kidney transplant recipients. Transplantation. 2011;91(8):858-63.
41. Heldal K, Midtvedt K. Managing transplant rejection in the elderly: the benefits of less aggressive immunosuppressive regimens. Drugs Aging. 2013;30(7):459-66.
42. Gill J, Sampaio M, Gill JS, et al. Induction immunosuppressive therapy in the elderly kidney transplant recipient in the United States. Clin J Am Soc Nephrol. 2011;6(5):1168-78.
43. Tullius SG, Milford E. Kidney allocation and the aging immune response. N Engl J Med. 2011;364(14):1369-70.
44. Pratschke J, Merk V, Reutzel-Selke A, et al. Potent early immune response after kidney transplantation in patients of the European senior transplant program. Transplantation. 2009;87(7):992-1000.
45. Hurst FP, Altieri M, Nee R, et al. Poor outcomes in elderly kidney transplant recipients receiving alemtuzumab induction. Am J Nephrol. 2011;34(6):534-41.
46. Moore PS, Farney AC, Hartmann EL, et al. Experience with deceased donor kidney transplantation in 114 patients over age 60. Surgery. 2007;142(4):514-23.
47. Debska-Sslizień A, Jankowska MM, Wołyniec W, et al. A single-center experience of renal transplantation in elderly patients: a paired-kidney analysis. Transplantation. 2007;83(9):1188-92.
48. Khanmoradi K, Knorr JP, Feyssa EL, et al. Evaluating safety and efficacy of rabbit antithymocyte globulin induction in elderly kidney transplant recipients. Exp Clin Transplant. 2013;11(3):222-8.
49. Heldal K, Thorarinsdottir S, Hartmann A, et al. Induction with interleukin-2 antagonist for transplantation of kidneys from older deceased donors: an observational study. Transplant Res. 2013;2(1):11-20.
50. Staatz CE, Tett SE. Pharmacokinetic considerations relating to tacrolimus dosing in the elderly. Drugs Aging. 2005;22(7):541-57.
51. Jacobson PA, Schladt D, Oetting WS, et al. Lower calcineurin inhibitor doses in older compared to younger kidney transplant recipients yield similar troughs. Am J Transplant. 2012;12(12):3326-36.
52. Bechstein WO. Neurotoxicity of calcineurin inhibitors: impact and clinical management. Transpl Int. 2000;13(5):313-26.
53. Besenski N, Rumboldt Z, Emovon O, et al. Brain MR imaging abnormalities in kidney transplant recipients. AJNR Am J Neuroradiol. 2005;26(9):2282-9.
54. Hanaway MJ, Woodle ES, Mulgaonkar S, et al. Alemtuzumab induction in renal transplantation. N Engl J Med. 2011;364(20):1909-19.
55. Woodle ES, First MR, Pirsch J, et al. A prospective, randomized, double-blind, placebo-controlled multicenter trial comparing early (7 day) corticosteroid cessation versus long-term, low-dose corticosteroid therapy. Ann Surg. 2008; 248(4):564–77.

56. Woodle ES, Peddi VR, Tomlanovich S, et al. A prospective, randomized, multicenter study evaluating early corticosteroid withdrawal with Thymoglobulin in living-donor kidney transplantation. Clin Transplant. 2010;24(1):73-83.
57. Tillmann FP, Quack I, Schenk A, et al. Prevalence and risk factors of pre-diabetes after renal transplantation: a single-centre cohort study in 200 consecutive patients. Nephrol Dial Transplant. 2012;27(8):3330-37.
58. Shah T, Kasravi A, Huang E, et al. Risk factors for development of new-onset diabetes mellitus after kidney transplantation. Transplantation. 2006;82(12):1673-6.
59. Luan FL, Stuckey LJ, Ojo AO. Abnormal glucose metabolism and metabolic syndrome in non-diabetic kidney transplant recipients early after transplantation. Transplantation. 2010;89(8):1034-9.
60. Burroughs TE, Lentine KL, Takemoto SK, et al. Influence of early posttransplantation prednisone and calcineurin inhibitor dosages on the incidence of new-onset diabetes. Clin J Am Soc Nephrol. 2007;2(3):517-23.
61. Duclos A, Flechner LM, Faiman C, et al. Post-transplant diabetes mellitus: risk reduction strategies in the elderly. Drugs Aging. 2006;23(10):781-93.
62. Trouillhet I, Benito N, Cervera C, et al. Influence of age in renal transplant infections: cases and controls study. Transplantation. 2005;80(7):989-92.
63. Dharnidharka VR, Caillard S, Agodoa LY, et al. Infection frequency and profile in different age groups of kidney transplant recipients. Transplantation. 2006;81(12):1662-7.
64. Parasuraman R, Abouljoud M, Jacobsen G, et al. Increasing trend in infection-related death-censored graft failure in renal transplantation. Transplantation. 2012;91(1):94-9.
65. Farrugia D, Mahboob S, Cheshire J, et al. Malignancy-related mortality following kidney transplantation is common. Kidney Int. 2014;85(6):1395-403.
66. Clarke CA, Morton LM, Lynch C, et al. Risk of lymphoma subtypes after solid organ transplantation in the United States. Br J Cancer. 2013;109(1):280-88.
67. Caillard S, Agodoa LY, Bohen EM, et al. Myeloma, Hodgkin disease, and lymphoid leukemia after renal transplantation: characteristics, risk factors and prognosis. Transplantation. 2006;81(6):888-95.
68. Dempster NJ, Ceresa CD, Aitken E, et al. Outcomes following renal transplantation in older people: a retrospective cohort study. BMC Geriatr. 2013;13:79.
69. McAdams-DeMarco MA, Law A, Salter ML, et al. Frailty and early hospital readmission after kidney transplantation. Am J Transplant. 2013;13(8):2091-5.
70. Grams ME, McAdams Demarco MA, et al. Recipient age and time spent hospitalized in the year before and after kidney transplantation. Transplantation. 2012;94(7):750-56.
71. Cornella C, Brustia M, Lazzarich E, et al. Quality of life in renal transplant patients over 60 years of age. Transplant Proc. 2008;40(6):1865-6.
72. Humar A, Denny R, Matas AJ, et al. Graft and quality of life outcomes in older recipients of a kidney transplant. Exp Clin Transplant. 2003;1(2):69-72.
73. Kniepeiss D, Wagner D, Pienaar S, et al. Solid organ transplantation: technical progress meets human dignity: a review of the literature considering elderly patients' health related quality of life following transplantation. Ageing Res Rev. 2012;11(1):181-7.

CHAPTER

7

Kidney Transplants in Individuals Infected with HIV

Pallavi Patri, Thangamani Muthukumar

ABSTRACT

Although highly active antiretroviral therapy (HAART) has had a dramatic positive impact on the survival of HIV-infected individuals, the prevalence of kidney disease among individuals infected with HIV is increasing. With regards to renal transplantation, the understandable reluctance to use immunosuppressive therapy in patients with HIV and the striking disparity between organ supply and demand have functioned to restrain organ transplantation in this patient population. Fortunately, renal transplantation for carefully selected HIV-infected recipients has become a reality. Major challenges exist in the management of HIV-infected organ graft recipients, in particular, a high incidence of acute rejection and the difficulties in managing therapeutic concentrations of calcineurin inhibitors in the context of drugs administered to control HIV replication.

HISTORICAL PERSPECTIVE

Historically, human immunodeficiency virus (HIV) infection was considered an absolute contraindication to kidney transplantation due to concerns that post-transplantation immunosuppression would put the already immunocompromised HIV-infected individuals at an increased risk for developing opportunistic infections and accelerate progression to acquired immunodeficiency syndrome (AIDS). Furthermore, in the pre-highly active antiretroviral therapy (HAART) era, allocation of organs to HIV-infected patients who experienced shorter life expectancy was considered wasteful of scarce donor organs.[1] Indeed, published experience from the 1980s of HIV-infected individuals who received kidney transplantations showed a significantly higher risk of infections including recurrent localized herpes simplex infections, candida infections as well as death from systemic fungal, bacterial and cytomegalovirus infections. A higher rate of acute rejection was also documented in HIV positive kidney transplant recipients.[2] Over the past two decades however, there have been considerable advances in the treatment of HIV infection resulting in significant improvement in long-term survival of infected patients. The HAART era that began in 1996 permanently changed the face of HIV infection from being a fatal disease to a chronic illness. As a result, there is less death associated with progression of HIV to AIDS. Instead, as individuals infected with HIV continue to live longer, morbidity and mortality from other chronic illnesses such as heart, liver, and kidney diseases has increased.[3,4] In the United States, HIV-associated nephropathy has now become the third most common cause of end-stage renal disease (ESRD) among black adults.[5,6] Understandably, there was initial reluctance to transplant individuals infected with HIV. However, thoughtful reconsiderations of the risks involved have resulted in a welcome foray into providing kidney allografts to HIV-infected patients.[7]

KIDNEY DISEASES IN PATIENTS INFECTED WITH HIV

Chronic kidney disease among patients infected with HIV may be a result of the viral infection itself as with HIV-associated nephropathy (HIVAN), immune complex disease associated with the HIV infection, treatment-related effects, or due to various virus independent factors such as diabetes, hypertension, or coinfection with hepatitis B virus or hepatitis C virus. Analysis of data from the Scientific Registry of Transplant Recipients (SRTR) revealed that from 1996 to 2009, hypertension was listed as the cause of ESRD in 39% of individuals with HIV, HIVAN in 14%, glomerulonephritis in 12%, diabetes in 10%, and others/unknown in 24%.[8]

HIV Associated Nephropathy

HIV-associated nephropathy is characterized histologically by collapsing focal segmental glomerular sclerosis with tubular microcysts and interstitial inflammation. HIV has been found to directly infect glomerular and tubular cells and induce epithelial cell dedifferentiation and proliferation.[9,10] HIVAN is usually associated with advanced viral infection and individuals typically present with nephrotic range proteinuria, enlarged kidneys, and advanced renal failure with a rapidly progressive course.[11–14] It is predominantly seen in individuals of African descent. Linkage disequilibrium studies have identified polymorphisms within the apolipoprotein 1 gene (Apol1) that have been associated with the development of focal segmental glomerulosclerosis and are found exclusively in the patients of African descent. These mutations are thought to confer resistance against trypanosomal infection that results in African sleeping sickness, which may explain the racial disparity seen.[15] It is unclear how these mutations in Apol1 may be related to the development of kidney disease, but it is associated with decreased expression of the gene product in podocytes and renal arterioles.[16]

Immune Complex Kidney Disease

While HIVAN remains the most common glomerular lesion in HIV-infected patients, up to 40% of patients who are thought to have HIVAN have an alternative histological diagnosis to explain their proteinuric renal disease.[17]

Several different immune complex-mediated causes of glomerulonephritis have been identified in HIV-infected patients including IgA nephropathy (IgAN), membranoproliferative glomerulonephritis (MPGN), membranous nephropathy (MN), "lupus-like" nephropathy, and immunotactoid nephropathy. Renal biopsy studies from the United States and across the world indicate that HIV-associated immune complex glomerulonephritis may be more common among Caucasian patients as compared to those of African descent.[11,18–21] In a multicenter retrospective study conducted in the United States, about 50% of HIV-infected patients who underwent renal biopsies were found to have diagnoses other than HIVAN including IgAN, MN, MPGN, and other immune complex glomerulonephritides. These patients were had less advanced HIV infection, were more likely to be Caucasian, and were noted to have a slower progression to ESRD regardless of HIV treatment.[19] There are several reports of HIV-infected patients with "lupus like" features on biopsy characterized by focal and diffuse proliferative glomerulonephritis and immunofluorescence positive for C1q, IgG, IgM, IgA, C3, lambda, and kappa deposits. Unlike other forms of HIV associated immune complex disease, this form of glomerulonephritis was associated with African descent and is manifested by a more aggressive course.[22]

Antiretroviral Therapy and Chronic Kidney Disease

Nephrotoxicity has been reported in association with antiretrovirals (ARV) in particular with the nucleoside reverse transcription inhibitor, tenofovir. Proximal tubular dysfunction with Fanconi's syndrome, nephrogenic diabetes insipidus and acute kidney injury as a result of tubular toxicity are well-described effects of tenofovir.[23] Whether tenofovir results in chronic kidney disease has not been well-established. A meta-analysis of 17 studies found that tenofovir treated patients did have a statistically significant loss of renal function as compared to those patients not treated with tenofovir, with a mean difference of 3.92 cc/min in calculated creatinine clearance. However, the risk for chronic kidney disease and ESRD did not significantly differ between the two groups.[24]

HIV and Hepatitis C Virus Coinfection

Hepatitis C infection is an important disease modifier in persons infected with HIV. When either infection occurs alone, during the chronic phase of the infection, a relatively stable viral load is maintained. However during combined infection, hepatitis C viral load increases after HIV seroconversion.[25] The characteristic kidney disease in patients with hepatitis C virus infection is cryoglobulinemic MPGN. Hepatitis C virus coinfection in HIV patients is common, affecting approximately 30% of HIV-infected patients. Multiple case series have identified HIV-infected patients with HCV coinfection who have glomerular diseases on biopsy including MPGN with or without associated cryoglobulinemia, fibrillary, and immunotactoid glomerulopathy. A large proportion of patients infected with HIV who have glomerular diseases are coinfected with hepatitis C virus.[26] There are limited studies that have focused on the treatment of the coinfected patients. The available data suggests that these patients may have a worse prognosis of their kidney disease than those infected with hepatitis C virus alone.[19,27]

PATHOPHYSIOLOGY OF HIV INFECTION AND IMPACT OF IMMUNOSUPPRESSION

Phases of HIV Infection

Human immunodeficiency virus targets both the innate as well as the adaptive immune systems. During initial acute HIV infection, the virus usually enters the host via the anogenital, tonsillar, adenoid, or intestinal mucosa where its viral envelope protein (CP-120) binds CD4 and CCR5 proteins on dendritic cells to gain entry.[28] This initial infection leads to recruitment of inflammatory cells and proinflammatory cytokines including IL-6, IL-18, and tumor necrosis factor.[29] Infected cells fuse with $CD4^+/CCR5^+$ T cells resulting in depletion of these lymphocytes particularly in the gut associated lymphatic tissue (GALT) and rising viremia with spread of the virus from mucosa to regional lymph nodes usually within 2 days of initial infection and into plasma within 3 days.[28] In conjunction with this viral spread, anti-inflammatory cytokines such as IL10 and transforming growth factor-beta (TGF-beta) are produced by the host immune system in an attempt to suppress the inflammatory response.[30]

These events lead to a chronically activated immune system characterized by increased T-cell expression of CD38, HLA-DR, Fas and multiple other molecules. Several other facets of the adaptive immunity are thought to be involved in the chronic inflammatory process that underlies the tissue damage seen in HIV-infected individuals. Gut mucosal barrier disruption that leads to translocation of microbial products may contribute to the chronic immune activation.[31] Additionally, antibodies to infected cells are produced resulting in binding that causes complement activation and deposition.[32] As memory CD4 cells become activated, they express CCR5 on their surfaces and thus become additional targets for viral infection, thereby perpetuating the chronic immune activation.[33]

Impact of Immunosuppression on HIV Replication and Infection

Cyclosporine

Several studies have highlighted the importance of cyclophilin A in the replication and infectivity of HIV.[34-36] The Gag polyprotein of HIV-1 is a polyprotein that is involved in multiple steps of the HIV viral life cycle.[36] On infection of a host cell, these retroviral polyproteins bind with and incorporate cyclophilin A into new immature virions. Cyclophilin A is thought to be required to destabilize the retroviral mature capsid prior to reverse transcription of viral products.[36] Cyclosporine A, a calcineurin inhibitor that binds cyclophilin A and suppresses IL-2-mediated T-cell replication, is commonly used as part of maintenance immunosuppression regimen in renal transplant patients. Cyclosporine A has been shown to decrease HIV infectivity and replication in chronically infected cells.[37] The clinical effectiveness of cyclosporine A as an adjunct to HAART in patients with acute and early HIV infection has been tested with varying results. In a study comparing treatment with cyclosporine A and HAART in patients with primary HIV-1 infection compared to patients treated with HAART alone, patients on combined cyclosporine A and HAART treatment were noted to have comparable viral suppression but higher $CD4^-$ T-cell levels than in the HAART alone cohort after 48 weeks.[38] A randomized control trial of 48 patients with acute and early HIV infection, however, failed to show any differences in HIV levels and CD4 counts between patients treated with HAART alone and those treated with combined cyclosporine A and HAART.[39]

Tacrolimus

Tacrolimus is another calcineurin inhibitor that is frequently used as part of the post-transplant immunosuppressive regimen. Tacrolimus, unlike cyclosporine, does not bind cyclophilin A. It complexes with FK-binding protein that then binds with and inhibits the function of calcineurin, thereby interfering with IL-2-mediated T-cell proliferation. Unlike cyclosporine, tacrolimus has not been shown to interact with the HIV gag polyprotein and does not appear to be involved in initial HIV infection; however, tacrolimus has been shown to interfere with growth of chronically infected cells and therefore viral production.[40]

Sirolimus

There has been interest surrounding the impact of sirolimus on the suppression of HIV replication. Similar to tacrolimus, sirolimus also complexes with FK-binding protein; however, this complex engages another intracellular protein called the target of rapamycin (TOR) as opposed to calcineurin. Inhibition of TOR leads to suppression of cytokine-mediated T-cell proliferation. In vitro studies indicate that sirolimus results in the downregulation of the CCR5 receptor and suppression of HIV replication.[41,42] Additionally, sirolimus was found to further enhance the antiviral activity of the CCR5 antagonist, vicriviroc.[43]

CCR5 inhibitors

Macrophage-tropic strains of HIV require the presence of CCR5 on host cells to gain entry and initiate replication. Homozygous mutations involving a 32 bp deletion in the CCR5 gene that has been identified in about 1% of the Caucasian population has been linked to resistance to HIV-1 infection, a decreased risk for the development of asthma, and a better course of disease in those with rheumatoid arthritis and multiple sclerosis.[44–46] During episodes of acute and chronic renal transplant rejection, CCR5 ligands are upregulated and the graft is infiltrated with CCR5 positive mononuclear cells.[47] Long-term allograft survival was significantly higher in a cohort of 21 kidney transplant patients who were homozygous for the CCR5 32-bp deletion than those who were heterozygous or had the wide-type CCR5 with a hazard ratio of 0.367 (95% CI, 0.157–0.859).[47] There are several CCR5 inhibitors that are currently being studied and one, maraviroc, is approved for the treatment of HIV. An NIH-funded study is underway that explores the possibility of using maraviroc in the prevention of graft-vs-host disease in those undergoing allogenic stem-cell transplantation. This drug class shows promise as adjuvants to the immunosuppressive regimen in transplantation in patients who are not homozygous for the CCR5 mutation in both HIV-infected and noninfected patients.

TRANSPLANT OUTCOMES

Patient and Graft Outcomes

Table 7.1 provides a summary of published studies on kidney transplantation in individuals infected with HIV. The studies reported thus far have shown good graft outcomes among HIV-infected individuals with ESRD who receive kidney transplantation in the current HAART era. The HIV-TR is the largest study with initial results published in 2010. This was a multicenter NIH-sponsored nonrandomized trial of 150 HIV-infected kidney transplant recipients followed for up to 3 years.[49] Patients received either antithymocyte globulin (32%) or Interleukin-2-receptor blockers (51%) or both as induction and were initiated on a steroid-based immunosuppressive regimen with either cyclosporine (22%) or tacrolimus (66%) and mycophenolate mofetil (MMF). Patient and graft survival rates were 94% and 88% at 1 year and 90% and 73% at 3 years, respectively. These rates are comparable to those reported by the US SRTR for all kidney-transplant recipients over the age of 65 years. Of equal importance was the finding that HIV infection remained well controlled as indicated by stable CD4 T-cell counts and few HIV associated complications. We reported from our center the outcomes among HIV-infected kidney transplant recipients maintained on an immunosuppressive regimen that included early steroid withdrawal.[48]

Table 7.1: Characteristics and outcomes of kidney transplant recipients infected with HIV

Characteristics	*Published reports*[*]											
Author	Stock	Tan	Kumar	Carter	Roland	Gruber	Touzot	Stock	Mazuecos	Muthukumar	Gomez	Gathogo
Year published	2003	2004	2005	2006	2008	2008	2010	2010	2010	2013	2013	2014
PMID	12883195	15591960	15780120	16539632	18093266	18645490	20840478	21083386	20858765	23503504	23622672	23970634
Number of patients	10	7	40	20	18	8	27	150	20	11	7	35
Males (%)	90	86	93	95	94	63	48	78	70	91	86	66
Blacks (%)	40	43	98	50	44	88	74	69	10	82	0	74
Age (years)	45 (median)	46±9 (mean ±SD)	46±6 (mean ±SD)	40–57 (range)	44 (median)	36–62 (range)	45 (median)	46 (median)	46 (mean)	53 (median)	45 (median)	40 (median)
Deceased donor (%)	60	57	90	60	56	88	93	68	100	73	100	56
Antibody induction	None	Alem 43%	Basilixi 100%	Basilixi 55%	IL2R Ab 39%	IL2R Ab 100%	Basilixi 97% ATG 3%	IL2R Ab 51% ATG 32%	Basilixi 30% ATG 5%	ATG 82% Basilixi 18%	Basilixi 43%	IL2R Ab 100%
Immunosuppression	CsA, MMF	Tac, Siro, MMF	CsA, Siro	CsA or Tac, Siro, MMF	CsA or Tac, Siro, MMF	CsA, MMF	CsA or Tac, MMF	CsA or Tac, MMF	CsA or Tac, MMF	Tac, MMF	Tac, MMF	CsA or Tac, MMF or azathioprine
Steroid maintenance (%)	100	57	100	100	100	100	100	100	100	0	100	100
Follow up, months	16.5 (median)	39 (median)	19.2 (median)	3.7–46.8 (range)	48 median	15 median	29 (mean)	20.4 (median)	40.4 (mean)	44.5 (median)	16 (median)	22 (median)

Contd...

Contd...

Acute rejection in year-1 (%)	n/a	n/a	n/a	n/a	52	12.5	15	31	n/a	9	40	37
Acute rejection total (%)	50	43	22	50	73†	12.5	15	41†	40	18	40	44
Infections (% of patients)	50%	0% (OI)	45%	ATG 55%‡ No ATG 22%	6% (OI)	50%	n/a	38%‡	30% (OI)	55%‡	0% (OI)	6% (OI)
Infections (total episodes)	5	0 (OI)	n/a	ATG 10‡ No ATG 2	1 (OI)	6	32	140‡	14 (OI)	8‡	0 (OI)	2 (OI)
Patient survival (1-year, %)	100	100	85	95	94	100	100	95	100	100	N/A	91
Graft survival (1-year, %)	100	71§	75	90	83	88§	98	90	85	91	N/A	91

Modified from Muthukumar et al.[48]

Alem, alemtuzumab; ATG, antithymocyte globulin; Basilixi, basiliximab; CsA, cyclosporine A; IL2R Ab, interleukin-2 receptor antibody; MMF, mycophenolate mofetil; OI, opportunistic infections; PMID, PubMed identifier; Siro, sirolimus; Tac, tacrolimus.

* PubMed, the MEDLINE (Medical Literature Analysis and Retrieval System Online) database maintained by US National Library of Medicine at the National Institutes of Health for articles published in the English language between June 1981 and January 2014 for kidney transplants in individual infected with HIV and who were treated with highly active antiretroviral therapy. Reports with five or more cases are shown in the above table. Reports from analyses of registry data are not included.

† Three-year cumulative incidence.

‡ Infections requiring hospitalization.

§ Graft survival during the follow-up period.

Results of this study revealed excellent patient and graft survival rates (100% and 91% at 1 year, respectively) with no progression of HIV observed at 24 months post-transplantation. Besides, urinary cell mRNA profiles among these individuals were comparable to that of kidney transplant recipients who were HIV negative and had stable allograft function with normal surveillance kidney biopsy results, suggesting molecular quiescence of the allograft.[49]

In a letter published in the *New England Journal of Medicine* in 2010, Muller and colleagues from South Africa reported outcomes of four HIV-infected individuals who received allografts from HIV positive donors. All four recipients maintained good allograft function and undetectable HIV viral loads at 1-year post-transplant.[50] This report created a worldwide debate on the ethics of such transplantation. In several countries, it is illegal to use organs from individuals infected with HIV. On November 22, 2013, President Obama signed the HIV Organ Policy Equity (HOPE) Act, into law that allows research on organ donations from individuals infected with HIV to another. This can eventually pave the way for HIV positive to HIV positive organ transplantation.

Interestingly, HIV infection has been documented in the allograft despite undetectable serum HIV viral loads. A recent study from France found that HIV could infect the epithelial cells of the transplanted kidney despite undetectable plasma HIV RNA levels in the recipient. In a cohort of 19 HIV-infected renal transplant recipients with undetectable plasma HIV RNA levels, 68% were found to have HIV infection in either podocytes, with podocyte apoptosis and loss of differentiation markers, or in tubular cells, often with abnormal tubular cell mitochondria. These findings were associated with a faster decline in allograft function and with subclinical acute cellular rejection.[51]

Acute Rejection

The NIH-multicenter study found a higher-than-expected acute rejection at 1 year (31% with 95% CI, 24–40) and 3 years (41% with 95% CI, 32–52), which was attributed by the authors to nontherapeutic exposure levels of immunosuppression. The study suggested the use of antiretroviral agents such as the integrase inhibitors, which does not interfere with the activity of cytochrome p450-3A enzymes to help achieve more therapeutic levels of CNIs and potentially reduce the incidence of rejection.[47]

Infections

A major challenge with the use of immunosuppression in HIV-infected kidney transplant recipients is balancing the risk of rejection with that of loss of HIV viral control and opportunistic infections. In the multicenter

NIH study of 150 HIV-infected kidney transplant recipients, those who received antithymocyte globulin in the first week had about twice as many serious infections per follow-up year as compared those who did not (OR 0.9 vs 0.4, $p = 0.002$). The study by Carter et al. specifically addressed the concerns of prolonged CD4 T-cell depletion with thymoglobulin use in the setting of acute rejection or delayed/slow graft function in their single center study of 20 HIV-infected kidney transplant recipients.[52] All patients were on antiretroviral therapy, opportunistic infection prophylaxis and maintenance immunosuppression with cyclosporine, MMF, and prednisone. None of the patients had received antithymocyte globulin as part of induction therapy, whereas 64% of those in the antithymocyte globulin group and 44% in the nonantithymocyte globulin group received basiliximab for induction. The mean CD4 T-cell counts remained stable in those who did not receive antithymocyte globulin; but, became profoundly suppressed in those who did. Despite adequate HIV control, CD4 T-cell counts took as long as 2 years to recover in some patients. There was no evidence of increased risk of opportunistic infections in those who received antithymocyte globulin; however, an increased risk of other serious infections requiring hospitalization was noted (10 serious infections in the antithymocyte globulin group versus 2 in the group that did not receive antithymocyte globulin). Rejection was successfully treated in all but one of the patients receiving antithymocyte globulin as evidenced by improved graft function and/or repeat biopsy with resolution.

Cancers

HIV-infected patients are at higher risk for the development of certain cancers. Exposure to chronic immunosuppression may further augment this risk. In the NIH-multicenter prospective study of 150 kidney transplant recipients, a total of nine neoplasms were reported. These included two cases of Kaposi's sarcoma, two of oral squamous cell carcinoma, two cases of skin cancer (one squamous-cell and one basal cell), two cases of renal cell carcinoma, and one case of thyroid cancer.[48] There were no reports of post-transplant lymphoproliferative disease among this cohort. The authors noted that aside from the two cases of Kaposi's sarcoma that were both treated successfully with sirolimus, the remainder of the newly diagnosed malignancies occurred at a rate that was comparable with that in non-HIV-infected kidney transplant patients. However, long-term follow-up showed a total of 14 neoplasms in 13 of the 150 transplanted patients occurring at a median follow-up time of 3.5 years post-transplantation. Thus far there have been three cancer-related deaths in the cohort.[53] The HIV-TR study further evaluated the progression of HPV-associated neoplasia among HIV-infected solid organ transplant recipients (either kidney or liver). There was an increased risk of developing high-grade squamous intraepithelial lesion among these patients regardless of type of organ transplanted or use of T-cell depleting agents.[53]

Overall, these findings of excellent patient and graft survival with good HIV viral control support the practice of kidney transplantation in the HIV-infected population as the preferred method of renal replacement therapy. The choice of induction therapy and appropriate treatment regimen in the setting of rejection will have to be further addressed. Data available thus far indicate that treatment of acute rejection as well induction with Thymoglobulin is probably safe. The risk for development of cancers in HIV-infected kidney transplant recipients is similar to that in noninfected recipients; however, studies with longer follow-up are required.

Issues in Patient Management

ARV and Immunosuppression

A major challenge in the management of HIV-infected transplant recipients is the interaction between antiretroviral medications and the immunosuppressive drugs commonly used post-transplantation (Table 7.2). CNIs and sirolimus are metabolized by CYP3A4, which is an isoenzyme belonging to the cytochrome P450 system in the liver. Several antiretrovirals either potentiate or inhibit CYP3A4, thereby affecting blood levels of these immunosuppressives.[54–59]

The clinical impact of these drug–drug interactions was reflected in the multicenter, prospective observational cohort study of 150 HIV-infected kidney transplant recipients who were followed for up to 3 years.[47] A higher than expected rate of rejection was noted at 1-year (31% with 95%, CI 24–40) and 3-year (41% with 95%, CI 32–52) estimates. The authors of the study suggested that these findings might have been a result of subtherapeutic exposure to immunosuppression. Though trough levels of CNIs were similar between the study population and those reported for non-HIV-infected transplant recipients, about one-third of the study cohort received CNIs less frequently than typically prescribed, raising the concern for overall decreased total exposure.[58] The kidney clears several of the antiretroviral drugs. Hence, dose adjustments are needed based on the kidney function. Moreover, drugs within the same class of HAART have different effects on the CYP3A4. Hence, simple rules of thumb for dose adjustments of CNIs while on HAART cannot be made. As several drug–drug interactions and dosing adjustments have to be taken into consideration while caring for kidney transplant recipients who are infected with HIV, antiretroviral therapy will have to be individualized for each patient. Close coordination between transplant physicians and physicians specializing in the care of individuals infected with HIV are essential.

Table 7.2: Potential interactions of HAART and immunosuppressive medicines

Antiretroviral drugs	*Effect of immunosuppressive drugs on antiretroviral*	*Effect of antiretroviral drugs on immunosuppressive drugs*	*Clinical effect*
Nucleoside analogs			
Stavudine (Zerit)	Antagonized by mycophenolate		Reduced stavudine activity
Zidovudine Retrovir)	Antagonized by mycophenolate		Reduced zidovudine activity
Nonnucleoside reverse transcriptase inhibitors			
Delaviridine (Rescriptor)		Increase CNI/ sirolimus	Increased risk for increase CNI/ sirolimus toxicity
Efavirenz (Sustiva)		Decrease CNI/ sirolimus	Increased risk for rejection
Nevirapine (Viramune)		Decrease CNI/ sirolimus	Increased risk for rejection
Protease inhibitors			
Atazanavir (Reyataz)		Increase CNI/ sirolimus	Increased risk for Increase CNI/ sirolimus toxicity
Darunavir (Prezista)		Increase CNI/ sirolimus	Increased risk for Increase CNI/ sirolimus toxicity

Protease inhibitors: The protease inhibitors, in particular ritonavir, are potent inhibitors of CYP3A4 and can significantly increase levels of CNIs and sirolimus. As a result, doses of these immunosuppressive medicines need to be adjusted when used in conjunction with protease inhibitors. In a study of HIV-infected kidney and liver transplant recipients, there were marked increases in cyclosporine, tacrolimus, or sirolimus trough levels that lead to either reduction in dose or increase in dosing intervals of these immunosuppressive medicines among those patients receiving protease inhibitors as compared to patients on nonnucleoside reverse transcriptase inhibitors (NNRTIs) alone or on no ARVs.[59]

Nonnucleoside reverse transcriptase inhibitors: Though the NNRTIs such as efavirenz and nevirapine have mixed effects on CYP3A4, they appear overall to be net inducers of this isoenzyme, resulting in decreased blood levels of CNIs and sirolimus. In the study of HIV-infected kidney and liver transplant recipients reported earlier,[58] patients on efavirenz and cyclosporine were noted to require much higher doses of cyclosporine than those on regimens without efavirenz.[59] Other NNRTIs such as delavirdine are potent inhibitors of CYP3A4.[60]

Nucleoside reverse transcriptase inhibitors: Most nucleoside reverse transcriptase inhibitors (NRTIs) are excreted via renal tubular secretion and dosing must be adjusted to renal function. They are not metabolized by the cytochrome P450 system in the liver.[61] This class of ARVs has been found to interact with MMF, which is a drug commonly used as part of maintenance immunosuppression post kidney transplant.[61] In vitro studies indicate that MMF may enhance the anti-HIV effects of the NRTI abacavir.[62] Authors of a small observational cohort study involving five patients with resistant HIV (defined as failing eight or more ARV regimens), uncontrolled viremia, and low CD4 counts reported reduction in viral loads with the addition of mycophenolic acid.[63] Further clinical studies are required to confirm these findings. MMF appears to inhibit the effects of other NRTIs such as the thymidine analogs, zidovudine, and stavudine.

CCR5 inhibitors and integrase inhibitors: Maraviroc, a CCR5 inhibitor, is neither an inducer nor inhibitor of CYP3A4 but is a substrate of this isoenzyme and thus has not been found to impact blood levels of CNIs of sirolimus. Drugs that impact the metabolism of CYP3A4 can have similar effects on blood levels of maraviroc as they do on CNIs and sirolimus.[8] Raltegravir, an integrase inhibitor, does not appear to have any interactions with other antiretrovirals or immunosuppressives.[8]

Opportunistic Infection Prophylaxis

In the HAART era, there is little evidence in the literature of an increased risk of opportunistic infections in the HIV-infected kidney transplant recipient over noninfected patients. Standard prophylactic measures that are used in the HIV-infected patients should be followed based on CD4 counts. Additional transplant specific prophylaxis guidelines particular to HIV-infected patients are listed in Table 7.3.[64]

GUIDELINES ON PATIENT SELECTION FOR TRANSPLANT

HIV-infected patients are required to undergo the same evaluation to determine candidacy for kidney transplant as noninfected patients. Additionally, several other criteria that relate to the patient's HIV status are scrutinized (Table 7.4). The cooperative clinical trials in adult transplantation (CCTAT) is a NIH-supported multicenter group that has put together practice guidelines for patient selection for solid organ transplantation.[64] The eligibility criteria for potential HIV-infected kidney transplant recipients as outlined by the CCTAT include CD4 count >200 cells/mm^3 for the prior 6 months, HIV-1 RNA load <50 copies/mL for 3 months with the use of a stable ARV regimen (or able to maintain a persistently undetectable viral load with the

Table 7.3: Prophylaxis for opportunistic infections in kidney transplant recipients infected with HIV

Opportunistic infection	*First-line medicine(s)*	*Alternative medicine(s)*	*Primary prophylaxis*
Pneumocystis jiroveci	Trimethoprim-sulfamethoxazole [1 double strength tablet (160 mg trimethoprim/800 mg sulfamethoxazole) or 1 single strength tablet (80 mg trimethoprim/400 mg sulfamethoxazole) daily]	Dapsone 100 mg daily, or Atovaquone 1500 mg daily, or Aerosolized pentamidine 300 mg monthly	Indicated in all patients for life immediately after transplantation
Toxoplasmosis	Trimethoprim-sulfamethoxazole [1 double strength tablet (160 mg trimethoprim/800 mg sulfamethoxazole) or 1 single strength tablet (80 mg trimethoprim/400 mg sulfamethoxazole) daily]	Dapsone 100 mg daily + pyrimethamine 50 mg weekly + leucovorin 10 mg daily, or Atovaquone 1500 mg daily, or Atovaquone 1500 mg daily + pyrimethamine 25 mg daily + leucovorin 10 mg daily	If CD4 T-cell count ≤100 at anytime
Mycobacterium avium complex	Azithromycin 1200 mg weekly	Clarithromycin 500 mg bid, or Rifabutin 300 mg daily	If CD4 T-cell count ≤50 at anytime
Cytomegalovirus	Acyclovir 400 mg bid, or Valganciclovir 900 mg daily		Indicated in all patients for 1 year from transplantation
Candidiasis	Clotrimazole troches 10 mg bid	Fluconazole 100 mg weekly	Indicated in all patients for 3 months from transplantation
Epstein–Barr virus	Ganciclovir 1 gm PO tid	Valganciclovir 900 mg daily	Indicated in all EBV negative Recipient/ EBV positive donor for 1 year from transplantation

Table 7.4: Criteria for selecting patients infected with HIV for kidney transplant[64]

- *HIV specific criteria*
  - CD4 T-cell count >200 cells/mm^3 for past 6 months
  - HIV RNA <50 copies/mL for 3 months (intermittent elevations to 1,000 copies/mL, not persistent on more than two sequential measures, followed by undetectable levels are permissible)
  - On stable ARV regimen for at least 3 months, or persistently undetectable HIV RNA level (<50 copies/mL) without use of ARV
  - ARV medication regimen compliance
  - Absence of active opportunistic infection or neoplasm
  - No history of AIDS-defining opportunistic infection/neoplasm except drug-susceptible candida esophagitis
  - No history of chronic cryptosporidiosis, primary CNS lymphoma, PML, *Aspergillus*, pulmonary coccidioidomycosis, resistant fungal infection, pulmonary/extrapulmonary tuberculosis
  - No significant wasting (BMI >18.5 kg/m^2, no more than 5% weight loss in preceding 3 months)
- *Non-HIV specific criteria*
  - Meet standard criteria for kidney transplantation
  - Karnofsky performance status ≥70
  - No history of influenza or RSV in past 30 days
  - Substance use per local site policy
  - Inability of unwillingness to comply with immunosuppression and prophylactic medication protocol
  - Ability to provide informed consent

use of ARV), and no active opportunistic infection or neoplasm. Patients with a history of prior opportunistic infections and AIDS defining illnesses such as chronic cryptosporidiosis, coccidioidomycosis, pulmonary aspergillosis, visceral Kaposi's sarcoma, primary CNS lymphoma, or progressive multifocal leukoencephalopathy are not considered appropriate candidates, given the concern that these conditions may worsen in the setting of immunosuppression. Transplantation, however, can be considered in select circumstances such as drug-susceptible candidal esophagitis, past infections such as pneumocystis pneumonia occurrence on diagnosis of HIV infection prior to initiation of HAART or distant aspergillosis with radiological and clinical resolution.[8,58,64] Patients should have a karnofsky performance status ≥70 and should not be suffering from significant wasting. Patients coinfected with HIV and HCV or HBV require additional evaluation by a hepatologist prior to consideration for kidney transplant. Compliance with HAART regimen is required as is compliance with monitoring of HBV or HCV.[64]

CONCLUSION

With better understanding of viral kinetics, HAART-immunosuppression interaction and effective infection prophylaxis, HIV infection is no longer an absolute contraindication for transplantation. However, transplantation of HIV-infected individuals should be limited to centers with sufficient experience in managing such transplants. Close coordination between transplant physicians and infectious disease physicians caring for HIV-infected individuals is important. We can hope that the HOPE act will eventually pave for kidney transplantation becoming the standard of care for all individuals with ESRD who are infected with HIV.

REFERENCES

1. Boyd AS. Organ transplantation in HIV-positive patients. N Engl J Med. 1990;323(21):1492.
2. Rubin RH, Jenkins RL, Shaw BW, et al. The acquired immunodeficiency syndrome and transplantation. Transplantation. 1987;44(1):1-4.
3. Selik RM, Byers RH, Dworkin MS. Trends in diseases reported on U.S. death certificates that mentioned HIV infection, 1987-1999. J Acquir Immune Defic Syndr. 2002;29(4):378-87.
4. Fine DM, Perazella MA, Lucas GM, et al. Renal disease in patients with HIV infection: epidemiology, pathogenesis and management. Drugs. 2008;68(7): 963-80.
5. Monahan M, Tanji N, Klotman PE. HIV-associated nephropathy: an urban epidemic. Semin Nephrol. 2001;21(4):394-402.
6. Abbott KC, Trespalacios FC, Agodoa LY, et al. HIVAN and medication use in chronic dialysis patients in the United States: analysis of the USRDS DMMS Wave 2 study. BMC Nephrol. 2003;4:5.
7. Stock PG, Roland ME. Evolving clinical strategies for transplantation in the HIV-positive recipient. Transplantation. 2007;84(5):563-71.
8. Norman SP, Kommareddi M, Kaul DR. Update on kidney transplantation in HIV-infected recipients. AIDS Rev. 2012;14(3):195-207.
9. Bruggeman LA, Ross MD, Tanji N, et al. Renal epithelium is a previously unrecognized site of HIV-1 infection. J Am Soc Nephrol. 2000;11(11):2079-87.
10. Ross MJ, Bruggeman LA, Wilson PD, et al. Microcyst formation and HIV-1 gene expression occur in multiple nephron segments in HIV-associated nephropathy. J Am Soc Nephrol. 2001;12(12):2645-51.
11. Williams DI, Williams DJ, Williams IG, et al. Presentation, pathology, and outcome of HIV associated renal disease in a specialist centre for HIV/AIDS. Sex Transm Infect. 1998;74(3):179-84.
12. Lucas GM, Eustace JA, Sozio S, et al. Highly active antiretroviral therapy and the incidence of HIV-1-associated nephropathy: a 12-year cohort study. AIDS. 2004;18(3):541-6.
13. Bigé N, Lanternier F, Viard JP, et al. Presentation of HIV-associated nephropathy and outcome in HAART-treated patients. Nephrol Dial Transplant. 2012; 27(3):1114-21.
14. Lescure FX, Flateau C, Pacanowski J, et al. HIV-associated kidney glomerular diseases: changes with time and HAART. Nephrol Dial Transplant. 2012;27(6): 2349-55.

15. Genovese G, Friedman DJ, Ross MD, et al. Association of trypanolytic ApoL1 variants with kidney disease in African Americans. Science. 2010;329(5993): 841-5.
16. Madhavan SM, O'Toole JF, Konieczkowski M, et al. APOL1 localization in normal kidney and nondiabetic kidney disease. J Am Soc Nephrol. 2011;22(11):2119-28.
17. D'Agati V, Appel GB. Renal pathology of human immunodeficiency virus infection. Semin Nephrol. 1998;18(4):406-21.
18. Nochy D, Glotz D, Dosquet P, et al. Renal disease associated with HIV infection: a multicentric study of 60 patients from Paris hospitals. Nephrol Dial Transplant. 1993;8(1):11-19.
19. Szczech LA, Gupta SK, Habash R, et al. The clinical epidemiology and course of the spectrum of renal diseases associated with HIV infection. Kidney Int. 2004;66(3):1145-52.
20. Praditpornsilpa K, Napathorn S, Yenrudi S, et al. Renal pathology and HIV infection in Thailand. Am J Kidney Dis. 1999;33(2):282-6.
21. Casanova S, Mazzucco G, Barbiano di Belgiojoso G, et al. Pattern of glomerular involvement in human immunodeficiency virus-infected patients: an Italian study. Am J Kidney Dis. 1995;26(3):446-53.
22. Haas M, Kaul S, Eustace JA. HIV-associated immune complex glomerulonephritis with 'lupus-like' features: a clinicopathologic study of 14 cases. Kidney Int. 2005;67(4):1381-90.
23. Tourret J, Deray G, Isnard-Bagnis C. Tenofovir Effect on the Kidneys of HIV-Infected Patients: A Double-Edged Sword? J Am Soc Nephrol. 2013;24(10):1519-27.
24. Cooper RD, Wiebe N, Smith N, et al. Systematic review and meta-analysis: renal safety of tenofovir disoproxil fumarate in HIV-infected patients. Clin Infect Dis. 2010;51(5):496-505.
25. Thomas DL, Shih JW, Alter HJ, et al. Effect of human immunodeficiency virus on hepatitis C virus infection among injecting drug users. J Infect Dis. 1996;174(4): 690-95.
26. Praga M, Gutiérrez Solís E, Morales E. Hepatitis C-induced renal disease in patients with AIDS: an emergent problem. Contrib Nephrol. 2012;176:24-34.
27. Izzedine H, Sene D, Cacoub P, et al. Kidney diseases in HIV/HCV-co-infected patients. AIDS. 2009;23(10):1219-26.
28. Kahn JO, Walker BD. Acute human immunodeficiency virus type 1 infection. N Engl J Med. 1998;339(1):33-9.
29. Connolly NC, Riddler SA, Rinaldo CR. Proinflammatory cytokines in HIV disease-a review and rationale for new therapeutic approaches. AIDS Rev. 2005;7(3):168-80.
30. Benito JM, López M, Lozano S, et al. Differential upregulation of CD38 on different T-cell subsets may influence the ability to reconstitute CD4+T cells under successful highly active antiretroviral therapy. J Acquir Immune Defic Syndr. 2005;38(4):373-81.
31. Brenchley JM, Price DA, Schacker TW, et al. Microbial translocation is a cause of systemic immune activation in chronic HIV infection. Nat Med. 2006; 12(12):1365-71.
32. Stoiber H, Soederholm A, Wilflingseder D, et al. Complement and antibodies: a dangerous liaison in HIV infection? Vaccine. 2008;26(Suppl 8):I79-85.
33. Picker LJ, Watkins DI. HIV pathogenesis: the first cut is the deepest. Nat Immunol. 2005;6(5):430-32.
34. Wiegers K, Kräusslich HG. Differential dependence of the infectivity of HIV-1 group O isolates on the cellular protein cyclophilin A. Virology. 2002;294(2): 289-95.

35. Streblow DN, Kitabwalla M, Malkovsky M, et al. Cyclophilin a modulates processing of human immunodeficiency virus type 1 p55Gag: mechanism for antiviral effects of cyclosporin A. Virology. 1998;245(2):197-202.
36. Braaten D, Franke EK, Luban J. Cyclophilin A is required for an early step in the life cycle of human immunodeficiency virus type 1 before the initiation of reverse transcription. J Virol. 1996;70(6):3551-60.
37. Briggs CJ, Tözsér J, Oroszlan S. Effect of cyclosporin A on the replication cycle of human immunodeficiency virus type 1 derived from H9 and Molt-4 producer cells. J Gen Virol. 1996;77(Pt 12):2963-7.
38. Rizzardi GP, Harari A, Capiluppi B, et al. Treatment of primary HIV-1 infection with cyclosporin A coupled with highly active antiretroviral therapy. J Clin Invest. 2002;109(5):681-8.
39. Markowitz M, Vaida F, Hare CB, et al. The virologic and immunologic effects of cyclosporine as an adjunct to antiretroviral therapy in patients treated during acute and early HIV-1 infection. J Infect Dis. 2010;201(9):1298-302.
40. Briggs CJ, Ott DE, Coren LV, et al. Comparison of the effect of FK506 and cyclosporin A on virus production in H9 cells chronically and newly infected by HIV-1. Arch Virol. 1999;144(11):2151-60.
41. Heredia A, Amoroso A, Davis C, et al. Rapamycin causes down-regulation of CCR5 and accumulation of anti-HIV beta-chemokines: an approach to suppress R5 strains of HIV-1. Proc Natl Acad Sci USA. 2003;100(18):10411-6.
42. Roy J, Paquette JS, Fortin JF, et al. The immunosuppressant rapamycin represses human immunodeficiency virus type 1 replication. Antimicrob Agents Chemother. 2002;46(11):3447-55.
43. Heredia A, Latinovic O, Gallo RC, et al. Reduction of CCR5 with low-dose rapamycin enhances the antiviral activity of vicriviroc against both sensitive and drug-resistant HIV-1. Proc Natl Acad Sci USA. 2008;105(51):20476-81.
44. Hall IP, Wheatley A, Christie G, et al. Association of CCR5 delta32 with reduced risk of asthma. Lancet. 1999;354(9186):1264-65.
45. Zapico I, Coto E, Rodríguez A, et al. CCR5 (chemokine receptor-5) DNA-polymorphism influences the severity of rheumatoid arthritis. Genes Immun. 2000;1(4):288-9.
46. Sellebjerg F, Madsen HO, Jensen CV, et al. CCR5 delta32, matrix metalloproteinase-9 and disease activity in multiple sclerosis. J Neuroimmunol. 2000;102(1):98-106.
47. Fischereder M, Luckow B, Hocher B, et al. CC chemokine receptor 5 and renal-transplant survival. Lancet. 2001;357(9270):1758-61.
48. Muthukumar T, Afaneh C, Ding R, et al. HIV-infected kidney graft recipients managed with an early corticosteroid withdrawal protocol: clinical outcomes and messenger RNA profiles. Transplantation. 2013;95(5):711-20.
49. Stock PG, Barin B, Murphy B, et al. Outcomes of kidney transplantation in HIV-infected recipients. N Engl J Med. 2010;363(21):2004-14.
50. Muller E, Kahn D, Mendelson M. Renal transplantation between HIV-positive donors and recipients. N Engl J Med. 2010;362(24):2336-37.
51. Canaud G, Dejucq-Rainsford N, Avettand-Fenoël V, et al. The kidney as a reservoir for HIV-1 after renal transplantation. J Am Soc Nephrol. 2014;25(2):407-19.
52. Carter JT, Melcher ML, Carlson LL, et al. Thymoglobulin-associated Cd4+ T-cell depletion and infection risk in HIV-infected renal transplant recipients. Am J Transplant. 2006;6(4):753-60.
53. Nissen NN, Barin B, Stock PG. Malignancy in the HIV-infected patients undergoing liver and kidney transplantation. Curr Opin Oncol. 2012;24(5):517-21.

54. Frassetto L, Baluom M, Jacobsen W, et al. Cyclosporine pharmacokinetics and dosing modifications in human immunodeficiency virus-infected liver and kidney transplant recipients. Transplantation. 2005;80(1):13-17.
55. Vogel M, Voigt E, Michaelis HC, et al. Management of drug-to-drug interactions between cyclosporine A and the protease-inhibitor lopinavir/ritonavir in liver-transplanted HIV-infected patients. Liver Transpl. 2004;10(7):939-44.
56. Jain AK, Venkataramanan R, Shapiro R, et al. The interaction between antiretroviral agents and tacrolimus in liver and kidney transplant patients. Liver Transpl. 2002;8(9):841-5.
57. Kumar MS, Sierka DR, Damask AM, et al. Safety and success of kidney transplantation and concomitant immunosuppression in HIV-positive patients. Kidney Int. 2005;67(4):1622-9.
58. Harbell J, Terrault NA, Stock P. Solid organ transplants in HIV-infected patients. Curr HIV/AIDS Rep. 2013;10(3):217-25.
59. Frassetto LA, Browne M, Cheng A, et al. Immunosuppressant pharmacokinetics and dosing modifications in HIV-1 infected liver and kidney transplant recipients. Am J Transplant. 2007;7(12):2816-20.
60. Huisman MT, Smit JW, Schinkel AH. Significance of P-glycoprotein for the pharmacology and clinical use of HIV protease inhibitors. AIDS. 2000;14(3):237-42.
61. Izzedine H, Launay-Vacher V, Baumelou A, et al. Antiretroviral and immunosuppressive drug-drug interactions: an update. Kidney Int. 2004;66(2):532-41.
62. Margolis D, Heredia A, Gaywee J, et al. Abacavir and mycophenolic acid, an inhibitor of inosine monophosphate dehydrogenase, have profound and synergistic anti-HIV activity. J Acquir Immune Defic Syndr. 1999;21(5):362-70.
63. Margolis DM, Kewn S, Coull JJ, et al. The addition of mycophenolate mofetil to antiretroviral therapy including abacavir is associated with depletion of intracellular deoxyguanosine triphosphate and a decrease in plasma HIV-1 RNA. J Acquir Immune Defic Syndr. 2002;31(1):45-9.
64. Solid organ transplantation in the HIV-infected patient. Am J Transplant. 2004; 4(Suppl 10):83-8.

Considerations for the Management of Hepatitis C Positive Kidney Transplant Candidates and Recipients

CHAPTER

8

Meredith J Aull, Sandip Kapur

ABSTRACT

Worldwide, hepatitis C virus (HCV) infection is more prevalent in the end stage renal disease population compared to the general population, and is a risk factor for increased mortality while on dialysis. Patients with HCV infection derive a clear survival benefit from transplantation as opposed to remaining on the transplant waiting list. Compared to patients without HCV, HCV positive [HCV(+)] patients are at increased risk of death, graft loss, rejection, new onset diabetes, and other complications, and thus the population presents complex management challenges for transplant clinicians. Eradication of HCV has significant benefits after transplantation related to patient and graft survival, and reduction in post-transplant complications, therefore patients should be treated with anti-HCV therapy before transplant. For patients with evidence of viral replication at transplant, HCV(+) donor kidneys represent an important option to decrease time on the waiting list. Ongoing research is essential for improving outcomes for this complex patient population.

INTRODUCTION

More than 150 million people (approximately 3.3% of the worldwide population) are infected with Hepatitis C virus (HCV).[1] The prevalence of HCV infection in patients on hemodialysis is much higher, up to 12% in the United States,[2,3] and even higher in countries with higher prevalence in the general population [such as Egypt, where up to 42.2% of dialysis patients are HCV positive, (HCV(+))].[4] HCV(+) patients on maintenance hemodialysis have been shown to be at higher risk for short term all-cause and cardiovascular mortality compared to HCV negative [HCV(–)] patients.[3]

In recent years, much focus has been placed on assessing kidney transplant outcomes in HCV(+) recipients; a good proportion of these studies show that HCV(+) recipients have inferior patient and graft survival compared to HCV(–) recipients.[5,6] Fabrizi and colleagues performed a meta-analysis that showed that HCV(+) kidney transplant recipients have an increased risk of death (RR 1.79) and graft loss (RR 1.56) compared to HCV(–) recipients.[6] Despite the inferior outcomes, however, it is clear that kidney transplantation conveys significant patient survival benefit vs

Table 8.1: Factors impacting outcomes in hepatitis C positive kidney transplant recipients

Important factors
• Gender
• Age
• Ethnicity
• Immunosuppression regimen
• Donor hepatitis C status
• Pretransplant diabetes mellitus
• Presence of viral replication at time of transplant
• Degree of sensitization to HLA antigens
• Pretransplant interferon therapy
• HCV genotype
• Extent of pretransplant liver disease

remaining on the waiting list,[7,8] where HCV(+) patients face an increased risk of death, particularly from cardiovascular disease.[8]

HCV(+) kidney transplant candidates have a higher prevalence of type 2 diabetes mellitus (DM) compared to HCV(-) patients, and contribute to the increased risk of death on the waiting list.[7] HCV(+) patients with ESRD are also at increased risk for hepatocellular carcinoma (HCC); risk factors in this population include cirrhosis, Asian race, and history of alcohol abuse, as well as male gender, increasing age, and DM.[9] Forman and colleagues described characteristics of HCV(+) patients on the kidney transplant waiting list; of 354 kidney transplant candidates, 7.3% were HCV(+); HCV(+) patients experienced a longer wait for transplant, were more sensitized to human leukocyte antigens (HLA), were more likely to be listed for a repeat transplant, and were more likely to receive a deceased donor transplant (as compared to a living donor transplant).[10] As will be seen in this chapter, there are many factors that impact outcomes of HCV(+) kidney transplant recipients, as shown in Table 8.1.

UTILIZATION OF HEPATITIS C POSITIVE DONOR ORGANS FOR KIDNEY TRANSPLANTATION

The utilization of kidneys from HCV(+) organ donors for transplantation into HCV(+) candidates is driven by the risk of morbidity and mortality while remaining on the waiting list, along with the shortage of organs available for transplantation. This practice has evolved from use in select HCV(-) and HCV(+) transplant candidates to today's practice of limiting HCV(+) organs to HCV(+) candidates with a actively replicating HCV (as evidenced by a positive viral load). Analysis of registry data to assess the impact of utilization of HCV(+) donor kidneys found poorer patient survival, regardless of the recipient's HCV status, while only HCV(+) recipients experienced poorer graft survival.[11] Utilization of HCV(+) kidneys for HCV(–) candidates deemed to have poor life expectancy on dialysis (due to type 2 DM with complications, significant cardiovascular disease, or lack of dialysis access) led to poor patient and graft survival, causing a change in policy to use HCV(+) donor kidneys only for HCV(+) candidates.[12] Use of HCV(+) donor organs for elderly HCV(–) patients has also been shown to cause rapid development of HCV infection, liver disease, and infectious complications, leading to poor survival compared to elderly recipients of HCV(–) organs.[13] Currently, the majority of transplant centers limit HCV(+) donor organs to patients with active HCV, avoiding patients who have cleared the virus (i.e. are anti-HCV antibody positive with a negative viral load). In addition, centers avoid introducing an organ from a donor with a more virulent genotype (for example, would not give a genotype 1b organ to a patient with genotype 2). Despite the large number of HCV(+) patients on the waiting list that might benefit from receiving a kidney from a HCV(+) donor, there unfortunately remains a high discard rate of HCV(+) donor organs (2.6 times more likely to be discarded).[14] Sadly, this demonstrates significant underutilization of this important resource, since only 29% of HCV(+) patients transplanted during the same time period received a HCV(+) organ, and those that received a HCV(+) organ waited 395 days less than HCV(+) patients who received a HCV(–) organ.[14]

A multivariable analysis performed to assess the impact of HCV infection on kidney transplant outcomes included various combinations of donor (D) and recipient (R) groups based on HCV status [D-/R- (n=1,897), D-/R+ (n=59), D+/R- (n=118), D+/R+ (n=95)].[12] The analysis found that HCV(+) donor status had a negative impact on transplant recipient survival, regardless of the recipient's HCV status. Graft survival was worse in all groups where the recipient and/or donor were HCV(+); the most common causes of allograft loss were death with a functioning graft and chronic allograft nephropathy. Kucirka and colleagues also analyzed outcomes after transplant, and although survival of HCV(+) recipients of HCV(+) allografts was inferior to HCV(+) recipients of HCV(–) donor kidneys, the absolute differences in survival were small (2% lower patient survival and 3% lower graft survival at 3 years post-transplant).[14]

TREATING HEPATITIS C VIRUS INFECTION BEFORE TRANSPLANTATION

Strong evidence demonstrates that HCV(+) patients with an undetectable viral load at the time of transplant have superior outcomes to those with a detectable viral load.[15] Patients with active HCV infection have an increased risk of renal allograft loss and poorer graft function, as well as a higher incidence liver disease in the long term.[15]

The ability to clear HCV infection prior to transplant has traditionally been hampered by the limited treatment regimens [i.e. combination of interferon (IFN) and ribavirin] and their poor tolerance by patients on hemodialysis due to their adverse effects (in particular, the anemia induced by ribavirin). Some centers have utilized IFN or pegylated interferon (PEG-IFN) monotherapy in attempts to clear HCV infection prior to kidney transplantation, with varying degrees of success.[16,17] More recent introduction of protease inhibitors as a therapeutic option to be added to PEG-IFN/ribavirin, as well as the potential for using cocktails of oral antiviral therapies that target HCV, has led to renewed interest in developing regimens that may be effective and tolerated by the dialysis population. In France, four patients with genotype 1b who previously failed PEG-IFN plus ribavirin were given a regimen of PEG-IFN, renally dosed ribavirin, and telaprevir.[18] Despite mild anemia requiring escalation of erythropoietin doses, the combination was tolerated and led to clearance of HCV after 12 weeks of therapy.

Regrettably, having cleared HCV prior to transplant does not always guarantee sustained viral clearance after transplant. Gentil Govantes and colleagues found that almost 25% of patients with a negative viral load at transplant experienced post-transplant reactivation; this was associated with a higher risk of mortality compared to those who did not experience reactivation.[15] Importantly, patients with a negative viral load at transplant who had received pretransplant antiviral therapy had a lower rate of reactivation compared to those who did not receive therapy (13.6% vs 41.2%; $P = 0.052$).

Specific recommendations for treatment of HCV infection in patients with chronic kidney disease are available.[17,19] Patients should not receive a kidney transplant while they are actively receiving IFN therapy, or for 28 days after completing a treatment course.[17]

DECISION TO LIST FOR KIDNEY ALONE VS LIVER/KIDNEY TRANSPLANT

The degree of liver disease/cirrhosis is used to guide the decision to list a patient with ESRD for a kidney alone vs a simultaneous liver/kidney transplant. Due to the shortage of organs, Paramesh and colleagues studied outcomes in patients with or without cirrhosis (majority of with HCV genotype 1a or 1b) who underwent kidney transplantation alone. The study found that patients with compensated cirrhosis and a hepatic portal gradient <10 mmHg did well, similar to patients without cirrhosis.[20] The authors suggest that liver/kidney transplantation in this subset of patients may be an unnecessary use of a liver allograft that can be utilized elsewhere.

PROGRESSION OF LIVER DISEASE AFTER KIDNEY TRANSPLANTATION

Research to assess the progression of liver disease in HCV(+) kidney transplant recipients has been sparse. Recently, Kucirka and colleagues reviewed 6250 HCV(+) kidney transplant recipients to assess the risk of being added to the liver transplant waiting list after kidney transplantation.[21] This study found that only 1% of kidney transplant recipients were eventually added to the liver transplant waiting list. Although the risk of needing a liver transplant was 2.57-fold higher for patients who had received a HCV(+) donor kidney, the absolute rates were very low in both groups. In addition, analysis of causes of death in the kidney recipients showed that only 6.9% of deaths were due to liver disease. Risk of liver related death was higher, but not significantly so, in recipients of HCV(+) donor organs.

Another group studied liver histology in patients remaining on the waiting list vs those who received a kidney transplant.[22] In 44 patients who had multiple liver biopsies, 31 of whom were transplanted, progression of liver fibrosis was less common in the transplanted patients (23% vs 62% in the waiting list group), and 16% of transplant recipient biopsies showed histologic improvement compared to baseline.

MANAGEMENT OF IMMUNOSUPPRESSION IN HCV(+) KIDNEY TRANSPLANT RECIPIENTS

The development of newer, more potent immunosuppressive medications, has led to renewed debate over the management of HCV(+) kidney transplant recipients, particularly since HCV(+) patients may be at higher risk for acute rejection episodes.[5,23] Debates include the following: Should induction therapy be utilized, or is the risk of viral replication too high? And which maintenance regimen is better for these patients who are historically at higher risk for both immunologic rejection and new onset diabetes mellitus (NODM)?

Induction Immunosuppression

Sureshkumar and colleagues investigated the induction immunosuppression question by analyzing HCV(+) patients who received a deceased donor kidney transplant in the United States between 1998 and 2008.[24] Patients who received induction therapy were broken into two groups, those that received a depleting (n=1,859) or nondepleting (n=1,631) agent. Patient and graft survival were similar between the two groups, regardless of whether the patient received a HCV(+) donor organ or not. Acute rejection rates were similar within the first year of transplant (10.5% in depleting vs 11.5% in nondepleting), and the use of depleting agents enabled more corticosteroid withdrawal (68.6% of depleting group on maintenance steroids vs 92.9% of the nondepleting group). Limitations of this analysis include lack of data on patients who received no induction therapy, as well as lack of data about the genotype and presence/absence of a HCV viral load at the time of transplant.

Information about the use of rituximab (anti-CD20 monoclonal antibody) in HCV(+) patients is limited. A case report published in 2007 describes use of rituximab for the treatment of gastric cancer in a HCV(+) kidney transplant recipient.[25] The patient developed cholestatic hepatitis C with a high viral load, hepatic insufficiency, pneumonia, and died of respiratory insufficiency. The authors attribute the cholestatic HCV to the rituximab administration. Rituximab has also been used to treat cryoglobulinemia after transplant,[26-28] causing disappearance of cryoglobulin-mediated glomerular deposits.[28] Basse and colleagues reported seven patients with cryoglobulinemia in the setting of de novo membranoproliferative glomerulonephritis (MPGN) after kidney transplantation. Clinical improvement was seen in all patients (as determined by serum creatinine, proteinuria, and cryoglobulinemia); however, two patients developed severe infectious complications (disseminated fatal cryptococcosis and disseminated herpes simplex type 2 infection), which led to the center to reduce their protocol from 4 weekly doses of rituximab to 2 weekly doses.[27]

Maintenance Immunosuppression

Much of the data on the impact of immunosuppressive medications on HCV infection comes from the liver transplantation literature and from in vitro studies. Therefore, it is unclear whether this data can be extrapolated to kidney transplant patients. Generally, immunosuppressive regimens are chosen based on the patient's risk for rejection in combination with the comorbid conditions exhibited by the patient or those for which the patients may be at increased risk (i.e. for a patient at high risk of developing type 2 DM). It is important to consider the degree of liver disease, since this may impact the patient's ability to metabolize immunosuppressants such as cyclosporine and tacrolimus, leading to a need for more judicious dosing and monitoring. Data available about the potential positive and negative effects of the individual immunosuppressive agents, derived mostly from liver transplant and *in vitro* studies, are summarized in Table 8.2.

Due to the negative effects of corticosteroids on viral replication, there has been interest at some transplant centers regarding early corticosteroid withdrawal in HCV(+) kidney transplant recipients.[23,42] Akalin and colleagues compared a small number of HCV(+) patients (n=12) undergoing rabbit antithymocyte globulin (rATG) induction therapy and early steroid

Table 8.2: Potential effects of immunosuppressive agents on hepatitis C infection

Immunosuppressant	*Beneficial effects*	*Detrimental effects*
Corticosteroids[29,30]		Pulse steroids/treatment of rejection associated with: • Increased viral replication • Increased risk of acute hepatitis • Decreased time to HCV recurrence after transplant • Increased risk of graft loss
Cyclosporine[31–34]	In vitro effects inhibit HCV RNA synthesis and protein expression • ↑HCV clearance in combination with IFN	
Tacrolimus[35–39]	Better patient survival vs patients receiving cyclosporine	Increased risk of new onset diabetes after transplantation
Mycophenolate mofetil[40,41]	• Inhibitory effect of IMPDH inhibition on viral replication • Patient survival benefit for recipients of HCV(+) donor kidneys	

withdrawal to a control group (n=17) who received triple maintenance immunosuppression plus nondepleting antibody therapy (n=7), rATG (n=5), or no induction (n=5). Patients undergoing early steroid withdrawal did not experience an increase in acute rejection, infectious episodes, or liver function abnormalities.[42] Our own transplant center reviewed our experience with 31 HCV(+) patients receiving rATG induction and early steroid withdrawal with 603 HCV(-) patients who received the same regimen.[23] Patients undergoing steroid withdrawal were at higher risk for acute rejection and graft loss, possibly due to the higher percentage of repeat transplant recipients and thus higher degree of sensitization in the HCV(+) group. Interestingly, however, only 5% of HCV(+) patients developed NODM, an encouraging finding and important benefit of steroid withdrawal in this population.

COMORBIDITIES SEEN IN HEPATITIS C POSITIVE KIDNEY TRANSPLANT RECIPIENTS

New Onset Diabetes Mellitus After Transplantation

New onset diabetes mellitus is an important complication in kidney transplant recipients, occurring in up to 25% of patients by 3 years after transplant.[43]

Patients developing NODM are at increased risk of death (RR 1.87) and death-censored graft loss (RR 1.46).[43] Risk factors for NODM in the overall kidney transplant population include increasing age, African American race, Hispanic ethnicity, male donor, increasing number of HLA mismatches, HCV infection, body mass index ≥30 kg/m^2, and use of tacrolimus as part of the initial immunosuppression regimen.[43] A meta analysis designed to analyze the relationship between HCV status and development of NODM in the kidney transplant population reported an adjusted odds ratio for NODM in HCV(+) recipients of 3.97.[44] It has been postulated that the high incidence of NODM in HCV(+) kidney transplant recipients may be at least partially responsible for the increased risk of death in HCV(+) patients. Potential mechanisms that relate to the association between HCV infection and NODM, include insulin resistance, decreased glucose uptake in the liver and periphery, cytopathic effect of HCV on pancreatic beta cells, deceased hepatic glycogenesis, and viral replication.

An immunosuppression tailored to recipient risk may help to reduce the risk of NODM for HCV(+) kidney recipients, balancing the risk of rejection with the risks of developing NODM. Our own center has reduced the risk of NODM in HCV(+) recipients from 25% to 5% by utilizing an early corticosteroid withdrawal regimen (internal data), and thus far, patient survival is similar between HCV(+) and HCV(-) patients receiving this regimen.[23]

Post-transplant Histologic Changes in the Renal Allograft: Membranoproliferative Glomerulonephritis, Proteinuria, and Transplant Glomerulopathy

Several groups have reported an increased incidence of de novo glomerulonephritis [MPGN or membranous glomerulonephritis (GN)] in HCV(+) kidney transplant recipients as compared to HCV(-) recipients.[5,45,46] Development of de novo GN is associated with proteinuria and an increased risk of allograft loss. Histologic evaluation using electron microscopy is important, to distinguish between GN and transplant glomerulopathy (TG), which is described below. Clearance of HCV through administration of pretransplant IFN therapy reduces the risk of developing MPGN.[47] There is some evidence to suggest that patients who develop proteinuria related to de novo GN after transplant may benefit from treatment with ribavirin monotherapy.[48]

Transplant glomerulopathy is a histologic lesion characterized by duplication of the glomerular basement membrane. TG is believed to be caused by chronic antibody-mediated injury, which causes proteinuria, allograft dysfunction, and represents a poor prognostic indicator for graft survival. Interestingly, the lesions share similarities with those of MPGN. Baid-Agrawal and colleagues reviewed cases of TG from their institution, and found that these shared three overlapping pathways of injury, including antibody mediated rejection [C4d(+)], thrombotic microangiopathy, and HCV associated glomerular lesions.[49] TG cases in HCV(+) patients were associated with a more rapid progression to graft loss compared to HCV(–) patients with TG. Unfortunately there are currently no therapies known to be effective for TG.

TREATMENT OF HEPATITIS C VIRUS INFECTION AFTER TRANSPLANTATION

Interferon therapy is generally avoided after renal transplantation because it stimulates the immune system. Therefore, it reserved for patients with worsening hepatic injury on biopsy or clinically decompensating liver disease.[17] There is ample evidence that administration of IFN after kidney transplantation puts patients at significant risk for acute rejection and allograft loss.[50] In cases where therapy is needed due to the progression of liver disease, IFN monotherapy is currently recommended.[17] Use of the newer protease inhibitors are currently contraindicated due to the clinically significant drug interactions with calcineurin inhibitors cyclosporine or tacrolimus,[51–53] although these drugs are beginning to be successfully utilized in liver transplant patients with recurrent HCV despite significant side effects and challenges in managing the drug interactions.[54,55]

MONITORING KIDNEY TRANSPLANT RECIPIENTS WITH HEPATITIS C INFECTION

Due to the complexity and comorbidities associated with the presence of HCV infection in kidney transplant recipients, it is important to monitor patients closely for development of complications and progression of liver disease. The current recommendations are summarized in the following bullets:[17]

- Monitor liver enzymes monthly for the first 6 months after transplant, then every 3 months
  - Refer to hepatology if abnormalities
- Monitor for liver disease annually
  - Patients with cirrhosis should have annual abdominal ultrasound and alpha-fetoprotein
- Screen patients for abnormal glucose and development of NODM
- Monitor for proteinuria using a protein/creatinine ratio or 24-h urine collection every 3–6 months
  - If protein/creatinine ratio >1 or >1 g proteinuria in 24-h urine, consider allograft biopsy.

CONCLUSION

Hepatitis C infection is a poor prognostic indicator for both kidney transplant candidates and recipients. However, despite outcomes that are inferior to HCV(–) patients, HCV(+) patients derive clear survival benefit from kidney transplantation. HCV(+) patients present complex management challenges to transplant clinicians, due to the risks above and comorbidities such as NODM and de novo GN. When possible, HCV(+) transplant candidates should receive anti-HCV therapy prior to transplant in order to attempt to clear the virus, as this has significant benefits after transplantation related to patient survival, graft survival, and reduction in the development of post-transplant complications. Clearly, the HCV(+) population deserves innovative research into new therapies to eradicate the virus prior to transplant, and strategies to best manage these patients after transplant in order to maximize patient and graft survival.

REFERENCES

1. http://www.who.int/mediacentre/factsheets/fs164/en/, accessed December 28, 2013.
2. Finelli L, Miller JT, Tokars JI, et al. National surveillance of dialysis-associated diseases in the United States, 2002. Semin Dial. 2005;18(1):52-61.
3. Kalantar-Zadeh K, Kilpatrick RD, McAllister CJ, et al. Hepatitis C virus and death risk in hemodialysis patients. J Am Soc Nephrol. 2007;18(5):1584-93.
4. Khodir SA, Alghateb M, Okasha KM, et al. Prevalence of HCV infections among hemodialysis patients in Al Gharbiyah Governorate, Egypt. Arab J Nephrol Transplant. 2012;5(3):145-7.
5. Morales JM, Marcén R, Andres A, et al. Renal transplantation in patients with hepatitis C virus antibody. A long national experience. NDT Plus. 2010; 3(Suppl 2):ii41-6.
6. Fabrizi F, Martin P, Dixit V, et al. Hepatitis C virus antibody status and survival after renal transplantation: meta-analysis of observational studies. Am J Transplant. 2005;5(6):1452-61.
7. Bloom RD, Sayer G, Fa K, et al. Outcome of hepatitis C virus-infected kidney transplant candidates who remain on the waiting list. Am J Transplant. 2005; 5(1):139-44.
8. Ingsathit A, Kamanamool N, Thakkinstian A, et al. Survival advantage of kidney transplantation over dialysis in patients with hepatitis C: a systematic review and meta-analysis. Transplantation. 2013;95(7):943-8.
9. Henderson WA, Shankar R, Gill JM, et al. Hepatitis C progressing to hepatocellular carcinoma: the HCV dialysis patient in dilemma. J Viral Hepat. 2010;17(1):59-64.
10. Forman JP, Tolkoff-Rubin N, Pascual M, et al. Hepatitis C, acute humoral rejection, and renal allograft survival. J Am Soc Nephrol. 2004;15(12):3249-55.

11. Bucci JR, Matsumoto CS, Swanson SJ, et al. Donor hepatitis C seropositivity: clinical correlates and effect on early graft and patient survival in adult cadaveric kidney transplantation. J Am Soc Nephrol. 2002;13(12):2974-82.
12. Singh N, Neidlinger N, Djamali A, et al. The impact of hepatitis C virus donor and recipient status on long-term kidney transplant outcomes: University of Wisconsin experience. Clin Transplant. 2012;26(5):684-93.
13. Flohr TR, Bonatti H, Hranjec T, et al. Elderly recipients of hepatitis C positive renal allografts can quickly develop liver disease. J Surg Res. 2012;176(2):629-38.
14. Kucirka LM, Singer AL, Ros RL, et al. Underutilization of hepatitis C-positive kidneys for hepatitis C-positive recipients. Am J Transplant. 2010;10(5):1238-46.
15. Gentil Govantes MA, Esforzado N, Cruzado JM, et al. Harmful effects of viral replication in seropositive hepatitis C virus renal transplant recipients. Transplantation. 2012;94(11):1131-7.
16. Werner T, Aqel B, Balan V, et al. Treatment of hepatitis C in renal transplantation candidates: a single-center experience. Transplantation. 2010;90(4):407-11.
17. Kidney Disease: Improving Global Outcomes (KDIGO). KDIGO clinical practice guidelines for the prevention, diagnosis, evaluation, and treatment of hepatitis C in chronic kidney disease. Kidney Int. 2008;109:S1-99.
18. Dumortier J, Guillaud O, Gagnieu MC, et al. Anti-viral triple therapy with telaprevir in haemodialysed HCV patients: is it feasible? J Clin Virol. 2013;56(2):146-9.
19. Gordon CE, Balk EM, Becker BN, et al. KDOQI US commentary on the KDIGO clinical practice guideline for the prevention, diagnosis, evaluation, and treatment of hepatitis C in CKD. Am J Kidney Dis. 2008;52(5):811-25.
20. Paramesh AS, Davis JY, Mallikarjun C, et al. Kidney transplantation alone in ESRD patients with hepatitis C cirrhosis. Transplantation. 2012;94(3):250-54.
21. Kucirka LM, Peters TG, Segev DL. Impact of donor hepatitis C virus infection status on death and need for liver transplant in hepatitis C virus-positive kidney transplant recipients. Am J Kidney Dis. 2012;60(1):112-20.
22. Roth D, Gaynor JJ, Reddy KR, et al. Effect of kidney transplantation on outcomes among patients with hepatitis C. J Am Soc Nephrol. 2011;22(6):1152-60.
23. Aull M, Guerrero J, Afaneh C, et al. Results of Early Corticosteroid Withdrawal under rATG Induction in Hepatitis C Positive Kidney Transplant Recipients: Inferior Yet Improved Outcomes. Am J Transplant. 2013;13(S5):357-8.
24. Sureshkumar KK, Thai NL, Marcus RJ. Kidney transplantation in hepatitis C-positive recipients: does type of induction influence outcomes? Transplant Proc. 2012;44(5):1262-4.
25. Fabrizi F, Martin P, Elli A, et al. Hepatitis C virus infection and rituximab therapy after renal transplantation. Int J Artif Organs. 2007;30(5):445-9.
26. Basse G, Ribes D, Kamar N, et al. Rituximab therapy for de novo mixed cryoglobulinemia in renal transplant patients. Transplantation. 2005;80(11):1560-64.
27. Basse G, Ribes D, Kamar N, et al. Rituximab therapy for mixed cryoglobulinemia in seven renal transplant patients. Transplant Proc. 2006;38(7):2308-10.
28. Bestard O, Cruzado JM, Ercilla G, et al. Rituximab induces regression of hepatitis C virus-related membranoproliferative glomerulonephritis in a renal allograft. Nephrol Dial Transplant. 2006;21(8):2320-24.
29. Bahra M, Neumann UP, Jacob D, et al. Repeated steroid pulse therapies in HCV-positive liver recipients: significant risk factor for HCV-related graft loss. Transplant Proc. 2005;37(4):1700-702.
30. Magy N, Cribier B, Schmitt C, et al. Effects of corticosteroids on HCV infection. Int J Immunopharmacol. 1999;21(4):253-61.

31. Nakagawa M, Sakamoto N, Tanabe Y, et al. Suppression of hepatitis C virus replication by cyclosporin a is mediated by blockade of cyclophilins. Gastroenterology. 2005;129(3):1031-41.
32. Nag A, Robotham JM, Tang H. Suppression of viral RNA binding and the assembly of infectious hepatitis C virus particles in vitro by cyclophilin inhibitors. J Virol. 2012;86(23):12616-24.
33. Firpi RJ, Zhu H, Morelli G, et al. Cyclosporine suppresses hepatitis C virus in vitro and increases the chance of a sustained virological response after liver transplantation. Liver Transpl. 2006;12(1):51-7.
34. Inoue K, Yoshiba M. Interferon combined with cyclosporine treatment as an effective countermeasure against hepatitis C virus recurrence in liver transplant patients with end-stage hepatitis C virus related disease. Transplant Proc. 2005;37(2):1233-34.
35. O'Leary JG, Trotter JF, Neri MA, et al. Effect of tacrolimus on survival in hepatitis C-infected patients after liver transplantation. Proc (Bayl Univ Med Cent). 2011;24(3):187-91.
36. Wiesner RH. A long-term comparison of tacrolimus (FK506) versus cyclosporine in liver transplantation: a report of the United States FK506 Study Group. Transplantation. 1998;66(4):493-9.
37. Luan FL, Steffick DE, Ojo AO. New-onset diabetes mellitus in kidney transplant recipients discharged on steroid-free immunosuppression. Transplantation. 2011;91(3):334-41.
38. Burroughs TE, Lentine KL, Takemoto SK, et al. Influence of early post-transplantation prednisone and calcineurin inhibitor dosages on the incidence of new-onset diabetes. Clin J Am Soc Nephrol. 2007;2(3):517-23.
39. Vincenti F, Friman S, Scheuermann E, et al. Results of an international, randomized trial comparing glucose metabolism disorders and outcome with cyclosporine versus tacrolimus. Am J Transplant. 2007;7(6):1506-14.
40. Henry SD, Metselaar HJ, Lonsdale RC, et al. Mycophenolic acid inhibits hepatitis C virus replication and acts in synergy with cyclosporin A and interferon-alpha. Gastroenterology. 2006;131(5):1452-62.
41. Abbott KC, Bucci JR, Matsumoto CS, et al. Hepatitis C and renal transplantation in the era of modern immunosuppression. J Am Soc Nephrol. 2003;14(11):2908-18.
42. Akalin E, Murphy B, Sehgal V, et al. Rapid steroid withdrawal in hepatitis C virus-positive kidney transplant recipients. Clin Transplant. 2004;18(4):384-9.
43. Kasiske BL, Snyder JJ, Gilbertson D, et al. Diabetes mellitus after kidney transplantation in the United States. Am J Transplant. 2003;3(2):178-85.
44. Fabrizi F, Martin P, Dixit V, et al. Post-transplant diabetes mellitus and HCV seropositive status after renal transplantation: meta-analysis of clinical studies. Am J Transplant. 2005;5(10):2433-40.
45. Ozdemir BH, Ozdemir FN, Sezer S, et al. De novo glomerulonephritis in renal allografts with hepatitis C virus infection. Transplant Proc. 2006;38(2):492-5.
46. Cruzado JM, Carrera M, Torras J, et al. Hepatitis C virus infection and de novo glomerular lesions in renal allografts. Am J Transplant. 2001;1(2):171-8.
47. Cruzado JM, Casanovas-Taltavull T, Torras J, et al. Pretransplant interferon prevents hepatitis C virus-associated glomerulonephritis in renal allografts by HCV-RNA clearance. Am J Transplant. 2003;3(3):357-60.
48. Kamar N, Sandres-Saune K, Selves J, et al. Long-term ribavirin therapy in hepatitis C virus-positive renal transplant patients: effects on renal function and liver histology. Am J Kidney Dis. 2003;42(1):184-92.

49. Baid-Agrawal S, Farris AB 3rd, Pascual M, et al. Overlapping pathways to transplant glomerulopathy: chronic humoral rejection, hepatitis C infection, and thrombotic microangiopathy. Kidney Int. 2011;80(8):879-85.
50. Fabrizi F, Lunghi G, Dixit V, et al. Meta-analysis: anti-viral therapy of hepatitis C virus-related liver disease in renal transplant patients. Aliment Pharmacol Ther. 2006;24(10):1413-22.
51. Hulskotte E, Gupta S, Xuan F, et al. Pharmacokinetic interaction between the hepatitis C virus protease inhibitor boceprevir and cyclosporine and tacrolimus in healthy volunteers. Hepatology. 2012;56(5):1622-30.
52. Wilby KJ, Greanya ED, Ford JA, et al. A review of drug interactions with boceprevir and telaprevir: implications for HIV and transplant patients. Ann Hepatol. 2012;11(2):179-85.
53. Garg V, van Heeswijk R, Lee JE, et al. Effect of telaprevir on the pharmacokinetics of cyclosporine and tacrolimus. Hepatology. 2011;54(1):20-27.
54. Coilly A, Roche B, Dumortier J, et al. Safety and efficacy of protease inhibitors to treat hepatitis C after liver transplantation: a multicenter experience. J Hepatol. 2014;60(1):78-86.
55. Werner CR, Egetemeyr DP, Lauer UM, et al. Telaprevir-based triple therapy in liver transplant patients with hepatitis C virus: a 12-week pilot study providing safety and efficacy data. Liver Transpl. 2012;18(12):1464-70.

Monitoring and Management of the Kidney Transplant Recipients with Donor Specific Antibody

CHAPTER 9

Sean Campbell, Darshana M Dadhania

ABSTRACT

The presence of circulating antibodies directed against human leukocyte antigens (HLA), pre-existing or de novo, portends early graft loss following kidney transplantation. Recent advances in technology have allowed for evaluation of donor specific antibodies with in-depth precision but not without challenges. The clinical significance of low-level donor specific antibodies is still debated and the optimal timing and optimal type of therapy still remains unknown. However, it is clear that if left untreated, there is a high risk for graft loss at 3–5 years from the initial detection of anti-HLA antibodies. As the number of patients on the waiting list for a kidney transplant grows, it becomes more important to intervene early and optimize graft survival. In this chapter, we review the data on the clinical significance of anti-HLA donor specific antibodies and associated diagnostic and therapeutic challenges.

INTRODUCTION

Over the course of human development the immune system has become both sophisticated and elegant in its function. The central role of the immune system is to distinguish self from nonself, thus ensuring that one can fight off pathogens and protect oneself from abnormal growth or malignancy. It is in the setting of this environment that organs are taken from one individual and transplanted into another. The first successful kidney transplant was performed between two identical twins in 1954. Since then the field has advanced significantly with the advent of new technology for histocompatibility testing and development of more potent immunosuppressive medications. In the current era, kidney transplants between two unrelated individuals are performed worldwide. Furthermore, due to advances in immunosuppressive protocols, kidney transplants are now performed across ABO and histocompatibility barriers.

Donor-specific antibodies (DSA) were first identified in the 1960s in the setting of kidney transplant rejection. In a landmark paper, Patel and Terasaki observed that patients who had preformed "cytotoxins" had significantly inferior allograft survival.[1] Preformed "cytotoxins" or antibodies directed against human leukocyte antigens (HLA) in the recipient arise from prior exposure to foreign HLA due to pregnancy, previous organ transplants or blood transfusions. The complement-dependent cytotoxic (CDC) assay identifies preformed DSA and serves as a surrogate for pre-existing humoral immunity. Based on the early demonstration of poor graft survival (<20%) associated with a positive CDC test, the transplant community recommends a prospective negative CDC crossmatch with the donor prior to proceeding with kidney transplantation.

Kidney transplantation is the preferred mode of renal replacement therapy. It is associated with improved survival and better quality of life. Furthermore, the cost of managing kidney transplant recipients is lower than the cost of managing them on dialysis long term.[2,3] However, the half-life of an average kidney transplant is 13–14 years for a living donor and 10–11 years for a deceased donor recipient.[4] In most cases, a transplant recipient will require a second kidney. Currently, approximately 16% of individuals on the waiting list have a failed allograft and are awaiting a second transplant. Sensitized individuals (those with preformed anti-HLA antibodies) make up 25% of the current waiting list and may have to wait more than 10 years for a transplant.[4] As a result, management of anti-HLA DSA to maximize the life of the kidney transplant becomes an important goal for transplant physicians.

DSAs IN KIDNEY TRANSPLANT RECIPIENTS

A large cross-sectional study of kidney transplant recipients (n=4,144) from around the world demonstrated that 22% of transplant recipients tested positive for anti-HLA antibodies and 10% lost function of their kidney transplant by 3 years.[5] In this study, the presence or absence of pre-transplant DSA was not studied. Large single center studies have also demonstrated that the presence of anti-HLA DSA pre-transplant is associated with a significant increased risk of graft loss and may be linked to the presence of concurrent class I and class II DSA.[6,7]

A retrospective study of 258 kidney transplant recipients demonstrated that at a median of 5.6 years of follow-up, 9% of those with a DSA pre-transplant developed antibody mediated rejection (AMR) with a hazard ratio (HR) of 6.6 (P<0.001) compared to those without DSA.[8] Furthermore, the risk of AMR was greater in those with either class II alone or in combination with class I DSA and in those with DSA mean fluorescent intensity (MFI) >8,000. Not only is the risk related to the DSA strength, but others have found that the risk of AMR within 3 months of transplantation increases with a rise in MFI value at 2 weeks post-transplant.[9]

A meta-analysis by Mohan and colleagues evaluated seven studies of kidney transplant recipients with preformed DSA but negative CDC and flow cytometry crossmatch.[10] The presence of DSA increased the risk for

AMR (RR = 1.98; $P<0.0001$) and increased the risk for graft loss by 76%. Overall, the evidence suggests that the presence of preformed DSA with or without a positive crossmatch will have a detrimental effect on allograft survival.

Even though individuals without preformed DSA have a lower complication rate and better graft survival, they are still at risk for antibody-mediated injury. In a group of 189 first time kidney transplant recipients, the incidence of de novo DSA was 11% at 1 year and 20% at 5 years.[11] The risk factors for developing de novo DSA were younger age, deceased donor transplant recipients, sensitization history with non-DSA anti-HLA antibodies, and mismatches at the DQ locus. In this cohort, the risk of graft loss following the detection of de novo DSA was 9% at 1 year and 24% at 3 years. The incidence of de novo DSA and 10-year graft survival were studied in 315 Canadian kidney transplant recipients with no preformed DSA. Fifteen percent developed de novo DSA at a median of 4.6 years post-transplant.[12] The 10-year graft survival in those that developed de novo DSA was significantly lower (57% vs. 96%), and the development of de novo DSA was associated with nonadherence and DR mismatch. In this study, presence of de novo DSA was also associated with the presence of subclinical antibody mediated injury on protocol biopsies.

In summary, the presence of anti-HLA DSA preformed or de novo results in increased risk for AMR and graft loss. The risk may be greater in those whose DSA MFI values are higher and in those that have both HLA class I and class II DSA.

DSA MONITORING

Since the development of the CDC assay, there have been numerous advancements to the field of histocompatibility testing that have paved the way for DSA monitoring post-transplantation. The current assays allow one to identify the specific HLA target of the DSA and provide information on the relative strength of the DSA. It is important to remember that these solid-phase assays are marketed as qualitative assays, not quantitative assays. Currently, most centers agree that high level of DSA pre- or post-transplant is associated with poor outcomes. There is no clear consensus on the clinical significance of low-level antibodies and there are no data on how different clinical immunosuppressive protocols affect the natural course of the preformed or de novo DSAs and allograft injury.

Assay for Measuring DSA

Solid-phase antibody assays first appeared in the 1990s.[13] Two major advantages of these assays are the ability to test for DSAs without the need for fresh donor cells and the ability of these assays to identify the specific HLA target of the DSA. An overview of the principles of these assays is provided here.

The first generation of solid-phase assay was based on the enzyme-linked immunosorbent assay (ELISA) in which the HLA molecules are immobilized to the bottom of the wells of a microtiter plate. Recipient's serum containing the anti-HLA antibodies is added to the well and if there are antibodies present against the HLA target, they will bind. This complex is then incubated with a reporter bound counter antibody specific for human IgG. A positive reaction will occur when the substrate for the reporter is added, if the recipient has an antibody against the immobilized HLA antigens. In this assay, the wells can contain multiple different HLA antigens for either class I or class II and gives a readout of "positive" or "negative" for each well. In a second level of testing, each well can be coated with a specific combination of HLA antigens that mimics an individual cell. With the latter assay, you are able to calculate the percent panel reactive antibodies (PRA) and identify specificities for the antibodies.

The next generation of solid-phase antibody testing utilized microspheres (beads) that contain various combinations of fluorochromes. Each group of beads can have a unique ID based on the combination of the fluorochromes. Assays based on these beads can be divided into three groups. The first level of testing can be performed with screening beads that are coated with multiple either class I or class II antigens and gives a readout of "positive" or "negative", similar to the ELISA assay. In the second level of testing, PRA beads, each bead is coated with 2 HLA molecules from each loci, mimicking a cell. Class I (A, B, C) beads are separate from the class II (DR, DQ, DP) beads. The most sensitive level of testing is performed with single antigen beads (SAB) in which each bead is coated with a single molecule of either class I or class II HLA.

In these bead assays, the patient's serum is incubated with the beads and then the mixture is then incubated with a phycoerythrin labeled counter antibody that binds human IgG. The secondary antibody provides the signal for a positive reaction and the bead fluorescence identifies which HLA molecules are bound to it. The read out can be on the standard flow cytometer or the Luminex® analyzer.

The solid-phase antibody assays offer several advantages and some challenges. These assays identify antibodies that are specific for HLA and identify both complement binding and non-complement binding antibodies. As a result, the sensitivity of these assays is much greater than the CDC assay. Within the solid-phase antibody assays, the Luminex®-based assay is considered to be more sensitive than the flow-cytometer-based assay and both of these are more sensitive than the ELISA-based assay.

The SAB assays also have the ability to identify antibodies specific for a particular allele when multiple alleles are represented on the panel. As the technological advancements occur and the assays are further refined, we are able to ask additional questions such as: Does the IgG subtype matter? Are complement binding antibodies more informative of the outcome?

Not all IgG subtypes activate complement effectively. The ability of IgG to activate complement varies by subtype (IgG3>>IgG1>IgG2), with IgG3 exhibiting the strongest affinity. A recently developed bead assay for the Luminex® analyzer can identify the IgG subtype of the anti-HLA antibody. However, there are no studies that link the IgG subclass with high rates of AMR or other complications in kidney transplant recipients. Hönger and colleagues divided kidney transplant recipients by weak complement activity (IgG2 and IgG4) and strong complement activating (IgG3 and IgG1) and found no difference in rates of AMR.[14] Conversely, Loupy and colleagues recently published a large study of kidney transplant recipients stratified by DSA status and by the complement binding status using the C1q assay.[15] In this study, they replicated the prior findings that DSA positive recipients had a lower probability of graft survival. Furthermore, kidney transplant recipients that had DSAs that were also positive for C1q had the lowest graft survival. Unfortunately, the paper did not study the IgG subtypes of the C1q binding antibodies, which may have provided additional information. In contrast, measurement of C1q binding antibodies in the pre-transplant setting was not informative.[16] Clearly, more research is needed to delineate the significance of C1q positive DSAs.

Challenges in Monitoring DSAs

Even though the solid-phase antibody assays are an essential tool for monitoring kidney transplant recipients post-transplant, the assays themselves are marketed as a qualitative assay and not a quantitative. In fact the use of solid-phase anti-HLA antibody assays to test the sera of potential recipients is a national requirement for all transplant centers in the U.S. However, data generated from these assays at one center may not be comparable to the results at another center and data generated from lot X may not be directly comparable to the data generated from lot Y.[17] Additional challenges in the interpretation of these solid-phase assays are described below.[18]

To begin with each center uses a different signal threshold for what they consider a positive reaction. As recommended by the histocompatibility experts, each center should evaluate their data to determine at what DSA MFI threshold correlates with a positive crossmatch. Depending on the aggressiveness of the transplant center or the centers' clinical protocols for sensitized kidney transplant recipients, different MFI thresholds may be utilized for proceeding with a transplant.

The variability in the assays themselves may influence the results of the test. The density of the antigens on the beads can vary from lot to lot and therefore the MFI signal can vary.[17] In addition, the antigen source (native or recombinant), conformation of the antigen on the beads and the specific alleles on the beads may vary from vendor to vendor or lot to lot. Laboratories may use different read-out platforms that prevent one from comparing results of one laboratory with another. Therefore, challenges of the solid-phase assays include the lack of standardization of reagents, techniques and read-out platforms from laboratory to laboratory.

Furthermore, to say that one does not have a DSA suggests that you have knowledge about the serum's reactivity against the donor's HLA antigens at the allelic level. Generally, the donors are HLA typed at low resolution only and therefore the alleles of the HLA antigens are not known. It is possible that the solid-phase antibody assay does not contain the allele that the donor types for. In this case, you will not be able to rule out a DSA with 100% certainly.

Consensus Guidelines on Monitoring DSAs

Given the clinical significance of preformed and de novo DSA, the transplant group has developed some guidelines for the monitoring DSAs post kidney transplantation.[19] It is recommended that the DNA of the donor and the recipient serum obtained at the time of transplantation for crossmatch testing be stored for future testing. This will allow for future risk assessments based on newly acquired knowledge in the field. The recommendations for DSA monitoring post-transplantation are based on the immunological risk profile of the recipient. These are outlined in Table 9.1. All transplant centers should have some monitoring protocol for de novo and preformed DSAs. Furthermore at the time of any protocol or for-cause biopsy, the kidney transplant recipient's serum should be tested for DSA using solid-phase antibody assay.

PATHOLOGY ASSOCIATED WITH DSA

High titer preformed anti-HLA DSA can result in hyperacute rejection and is associated with cyanosis of the graft within minutes to hours. The histology of the graft demonstrates microvascular thrombosis, interstitial hemorrhage, tubular injury, micro- and macro-vascular inflammation and cortical necrosis. Fortunately, this is a rare event in the current era where all kidney transplant recipients are screened for high titer antibodies using the CDC assay. The more common pattern of injury associated with circulating DSA is acute and chronic AMR. The routine use of solid-phase assays to measure DSA and molecular evaluations of biopsies suggesting

Table 9.1: Post-transplant DSA monitoring recommendations

	Low risk	*Intermediate risk*	*High risk*	*Very high risk*
Group definitions	No sensitization history	Sensitization history and history of DSA historically	DSA positive and Crossmatch Negative	Desensitized
DSA test within first 3 months		DSA test; protocol biopsy if DSA positive*	DSA test and protocol biopsy†	DSA test and Protocol biopsy†
DSA test Month 3 to Month 12	At least once		Interval DSA monitoring‡	Interval DSA monitoring‡
After Month 12	Test for DSA if there is*: (1) significant change in immunosuppressive therapy, (2) suspicion for nonadherence, (3) graft dysfunction			

Adapted from Tait et al.[19]

*Level 2 recommendation.

†Level 1 recommendation to perform a biopsy and level 2 recommendation to treat subclinical AMR.

‡Level 2 recommendation to treat and/or perform a biopsy if there is significant increase in DSA.

that endothelial injury is present even in the absence of C4d staining of peritubular capillaries has resulted in further refinement of the diagnostic criteria for acute and chronic AMR.

According to the most recent diagnostic criteria, set up by the Banff Committee in 2013, diagnosis of acute AMR requires the presence of (a) histological evidence of acute tissue injury, (b) evidence of current or recent antibody interaction with vascular endothelium, and (c) serologic evidence of DSA.[20] In this revised classification, tissue injury can be acute tubular injury, any level of microvascular inflammation, thrombotic microangiopathy (TMA), or arthritis. Evidence for antibody interaction with the endothelium can be either the presence of linear C4d deposition in the peritubular capillaries or microvascular inflammation of grade 2 or higher. By eliminating the requirement for positive C4d staining, this revised classification resolves the controversy associated with the positive C4d requirement for AMR diagnosis.

Diagnosis of chronic AMR also has three diagnostic criteria: (a) histological evidence of chronic tissue injury, (b) evidence of current or recent antibody interaction with vascular endothelium, and (c) serological evidence of DSA. The latter two criteria are identical and therefore the main distinguishing feature of chronic AMR from acute AMR is the type of injury. In chronic AMR, there should be evidence of transplant glomerulopathy (TG) or multilayering of peritubular basement membranes or arterial intimal fibrosis.

Lastly, there is an entity called C4d positive staining without evidence of rejection. This entity is mainly applicable to protocol biopsies performed on ABO incompatible transplants, where the presence of anti-blood-group antibodies may not be injurious to the graft and the positive C4d staining may be a sign of accommodation. The presence of circulating anti-HLA DSA precludes the diagnosis of C4d staining without evidence of rejection.

The diagnosis of subclinical AMR was discussed in the Banff '07 meeting report. Data from that meeting suggested that 12% of individuals who were transplanted with strong DSA(s) will develop subclinical AMR and subclinical AMR was associated with a high risk of fibrosis and TG at 1 year.[21] Recent review of 1,101 biopsies demonstrated that the incidence of subclinical AMR was 8% and most of these biopsies had an incomplete phenotype (defined by the Banff '07 criteria).[22] They found the presence of DSA correlated with the presence of microvascular injury. A prospective protocol biopsy study of kidney transplant recipients with and without DSA showed that kidney transplant recipients who had DSA had increased risk for microvascular inflammation on their 3 months and 1-year protocol biopsies.[23] Furthermore, if the 3-month biopsy demonstrated microvascular inflammation with or without positive C4d staining, the risk of fibrosis at 1 year was significantly increased (100% in the C4d positive group and 77% in the C4d negative group with microvascular inflammation and 33% in those without these findings). Furthermore, the GFR at 1 year was significantly lower in both groups with microvascular inflammation and the incidence of TG on the 1-year biopsy was 43% and 18% in the microvascular inflammation groups with and without positive C4d staining respectively. The group without microvascular inflammation did not develop TG at 1 year. These data suggest that the changes in the diagnostic criteria for AMR set up by the Banff 2013 meeting are also applicable to the diagnosis of subclinical AMR. Microvascular inflammation is a key component of antibody-mediated injury in renal allografts and is associated with increased risk of fibrosis and subsequent decline in renal function.

MANAGEMENT OF DSA

Isolated antibody mediated injury is a rare event since T-cell help is required for a mature B cell response. Aside from a hyperacute rejection episode associated with high titer preformed antibodies, treatment of AMR requires control of the T cell response as well as the B cell response. As a result, almost all centers at the very least will use pulse steroids and escalation of maintenance immunosuppression as one of the components of therapy.[24] In addition, AMR requires targeted therapy for the existing circulating alloantibodies and the B-cell compartment (Table 9.2). The mechanisms of the B-cell targeted therapies are outlined below:

Table 9.2: Current options for treatment of acute antibody mediated rejection

- Decrease inflammatory response
  - Steroids
  - IVIG
- Reduce titer of circulating anti-HLA DSA
  - Plasma exchange/immunoadsorption
  - Proteasome inhibition
- Impair function of circulating anti-HLA DSA
  - IVIG
  - Inhibition of the complement system
- Impair B cell immune response
  - IVIG
  - Anti-CD20 antibody
  - Proteasome inhibition
  - Inhibition of the complement system

Intravenous immunoglobulin (IVIG): The effects of IVIG on the immune system are multiple. IVIG is believed to have neutralizing effect on the circulating alloantibodies, enhances clearance of alloantibodies, functions as a scavenger of activated complements, can promote apoptosis of B cells via signaling through the Fc-gamma receptors expressed on B cells, and suppresses inflammation through novel Th-2 pathway.[24] IVIG has been an integral component of many AMR treatment protocols.

Rituximab: Rituximab is a chimeric monoclonal antibody that binds CD20, a molecule that is present on naïve and mature B cells as well as some memory cells. Treatment with anti-CD20 antibody leads to B-cell depletion via antibody-dependent cytotoxicity. The effect of anti-CD20 antibody on circulating peripheral B cells can last 6–12 months.[25] Rituximab has been used as adjunctive therapy to treat AMR and may be beneficial by eliminating B cell function as an antigen presenting cell and as a plasma cell precursor.

Bortezomib: Bortezomib is a proteasome inhibitor that is used to treat plasma cell disorders. Bortezomib inhibits ubiquitin-proteasome pathway by binding to the 26S proteasome and promotes cell cycle arrest and cell apoptosis. In whole bone marrow cultures, bortezomib is able to selectively induce apoptosis of plasma cells.[26] Treatment with bortezomib is able to reduce DSA levels much better than treatment with rituximab. However, the effect is variable depending on the type of DSA and the strength of DSA.

Eculizumab: The latest therapy to join the armamentarium for treatment of acute AMR is the anti-C5 monoclonal antibody, eculizumab. It inhibits the final step of complement activation by inhibiting the cleavage of C5 to C5a and C5b, which in turn prevents the formation of the terminal complement complex C5b-9.[24] It is currently approved for the management of paroxysmal nocturnal hemoglobinuria and atypical hemolytic uremic syndrome. At the current time, there are limited data on the use of this therapy for treatment of AMR.

There are very few randomized controlled studies that focused on the treatment of AMR. The sections below review the current literature on the treatment of acute, chronic and subclinical AMR.

Antibody-mediated Rejection

The earliest studies on treatment of acute AMR utilized removal of the antibodies as the central component to therapy. In 1983, a study in France compared treatment with conventional therapy (steroids and azathioprine) vs aggressive plasma exchange (PE) with conventional therapy in a group of kidney transplant recipients with DSA who experienced early rejection episodes.[27] The antibody titer did decrease in the PE group but there was no difference in the graft function between the two groups over time. Since then, there were few small randomized controlled trials evaluating the use of plasma exchange for treatment of AMR that showed mixed results.[28] The most impressive results were seen in a recent randomized controlled trial that was performed with use of immunoadsorption – (protein A columns) to reduce the titer of DSA. They compared the conventional treatment of steroids and conversion to tacrolimus and mycophenolate mofetil therapy with the conventional treatment plus immunoadsorption in recipients with C4d-positive acute AMR. The trial was stopped early due to increased risk of graft loss in the conventional treatment arm. In a recent review of 8 studies containing 79 kidney transplant recipients who were treated with PE/IVIG for AMR, the graft survival and recipient survival were 82% and 98%, respectively, during a mean of 20-month follow-up.[29] In general, combination of plasma exchange and IVIG has been useful in the management of AMR and is associated with good short-term outcomes.

Jordan and colleagues described the use of high dose IVIG to treat 10 kidney transplant recipients with AMR in 1998.[30] In this cohort, 9 or 10 recipients responded to the therapy. For IVIG therapy, there has only been one randomized controlled trial. In this trial, kidney transplant recipients with steroid resistant acute rejection (not specifically acute AMR) were randomized to receive either OKT3 or IVIG.[31] Those treated with IVIG had lower rate of acute rejection recurrence and had comparable graft and recipient survival to those who received OKT3. Although the use of IVIG alone, even high dose, seems to be safe, most centers are using IVIG in combination with plasma exchange. In fact for desensitization protocol, low-dose IVIG with plasma exchange and rituximab outperformed high-dose IVIG alone.[32]

The data on the use of rituximab for treatment of AMR are also limited to case series and retrospective reviews. In a retrospective study by Kaposztas and colleagues evaluated treatment with PE alone (n=28) vs those that received PE and rituximab (n=26) for acute AMR.[33] They found that the 2-year survival was much better for the PE/rituximab group (90%) compared to PE alone group (60%). Multivariable analysis revealed that treatment with rituximab was the most important predictor of graft survival. Lefaucheur and colleagues compared treatment with PE/IVIG/rituximab with their retrospective cohort that received high-dose IVIG only.[34] They found that the group that received combination therapy had significant decrease in DSA and improved graft survival. Furthermore, the presence of high titer DSA predicted poor response and graft failure.

The proteasome inhibitor, bortezomib, has the potential to target antibody producing cells. Given that DSA reduction is one of the goals in AMR, recent treatment protocols have evaluated the effect of bortezomib therapy on acute AMR outcomes. In one of the initial studies, Everly and colleagues demonstrated that treatment with bortezomib in combination with other therapies was effective in reversing the mixed rejection associated with circulating DSA and improving renal function.[35] In a follow-up study, the same group demonstrated that 50% reduction in DSA associated with bortezomib-based therapy improved allograft survival.[36] Flechner and colleagues treated 20 kidney transplant recipients with C4d+ acute AMR with steroids/PE/IVIG and four doses of bortezomib.[37] Overall graft survival was 85% and they found that those with creatinine <3 and proteinuria of <1 g benefited the most. Recent retrospective review compared the efficacy of rituximab vs bortezomib-based therapy in kidney transplant recipients with acute AMR. All recipients received steroids, PE and IVIG. The 9-month creatinine and the 18-months graft survival were better in the bortezomib group.[38]

As antibody-induced complement activation is an important pathogenic pathway in AMR, the use of the complement inhibitor, eculizumab, is an intriguing therapeutic option. To date, there are only case reports describing the use of eculizumab to treat refractory AMR in ABO-incompatible transplants and in AMR associated with TMA.[39,40] In a small case series, the group from Mayo Clinic showed that with the use of eculizumab-based desensitization protocol, the rate of acute AMR was low.[41] At the present time, there are no long-term studies. This therapy may be helpful in the management of acute AMR but may not be optimal therapy for long-term management. Use of eculizumab as part of desensitization protocol did result in successful transplantation but it did not prevent chronic AMR.

Subclinical/Chronic AMR

With the acceptance of C4d negative AMR as an entity and the emphasis on the microvascular inflammation as one of the diagnostic criteria for AMR in the Banff 2014 meeting report, the definitions of subclinical and chronic AMR have changed significantly.[20] Now a kidney transplant recipient with circulating DSA and evidence of microvascular inflammation has by definition evidence of subclinical AMR. Previous protocol biopsy studies in high-risk recipients have demonstrated that the presence of subclinical AMR, as defined above, is associated with decline in renal function and development of chronic injury, diagnostic of chronic AMR.[42,43] At this time, there are no data on outcomes of treating subclinical AMR. However, based on previous studies of treating subclinical cellular rejection, one can extrapolate that there would be a benefit from treatment subclinical AMR. Data from acute AMR treatment indicates that reduction in DSA is associated with better renal allograft function. Therefore, it may be reasonable to target the DSA level when managing subclinical AMR on protocol biopsies. The optimal therapy to manage subclinical AMR and prevent chronic AMR requires further research and well-designed prospective trials.

Chronic AMR may be the result of persistent subclinical AMR and is the late manifestation of chronic immune injury. TG is the primary manifestation of chronic AMR and approximately 20% of kidney transplant recipients will develop TG by 5 years.[44] The risk factors for TG include acute rejection, preformed DSA as well as de novo DSA. Issa and colleagues found that the risk of TG was significantly higher in transplant recipients with Class II DSA.[45] Furthermore higher class II DSAs were associated with positive C4d staining on biopsy and both were related to increased risk of graft loss. In this study, the risk of graft loss was 38% in those with TG and 5% in those without TG during the follow-up period.

At the current time, prospective studies to evaluate various treatment protocols in kidney transplant recipients with TG are lacking. There is a small study of six pediatric transplant recipients who received combination of IVIG (1 g/kg) × 4 doses and rituximab (375 mg/m^2) × 1 dose at the time of chronic antibody mediated injury.[46] Four out of the 6 responded with improvement or stabilization of GFR at 12 months. The two non-responders had more extensive TG, C4d deposition and more inflammation on their initial biopsy. A similar pilot study of 6 adult kidney transplant recipients using rituximab (375 mg/m^2) × 1 followed by 4 doses of IVIG (0.4 g/kg) demonstrated that three recipients responded with improvement or stabilization of renal function.[47] The nonresponders had higher degree of TG, lower renal function, and more proteinuria at the time of diagnosis.

The above data suggest that early intervention may be more beneficial. A recent publication described the outcomes associated with the use of peritransplant rituximab in kidney transplant recipients with preformed DSA.[48] The cohort was divided into four groups as shown in Table 9.3. In the DSA positive group, those that received rituximab therapy had lower incidence of acute rejection and chronic AMR. Future prospective

Table 9.3: Prevention of chronic antibody rejection using rituximab

	DSA positive (N = 39)	*DSA negative (N = 121)*	*DSA positive (N = 74)*
Rituximab treatment*	None	None	200 mg + PE × 4
6 month acute rejection	39%	19%	15%
Chronic AMR	50%	22%	18%
De novo DSA	13%	12%	0%
5-year graft survival	84%	95%	98%

Adapted from Ishida et al.[48]

PE, plasma exchange.

*All received basiliximab induction and maintenance with tacrolimus, mycophenolate mofetil and prednisone.

randomized interventional studies that address preventive and pre-emptive therapy for chronic AMR will add to our understanding of chronic AMR management.

SUMMARY

Over the past two decades there have been extraordinary advancements in our understanding of how the immune response works. This has led to significant advancements in histocompatibility testing and development of novel therapeutics. Combination of these two factors are leading the way to the development of targeted treatment protocols and individualization of therapy to prevent chronic injury and improve the long-term outcomes of kidney transplant recipients.

REFERENCES

1. Patel R, Terasaki PI. Significance of the positive crossmatch test in kidney transplantation. N Engl J Med. 1969;280(14):735-9.
2. Evans RW, Manninen DL, Garrison LP, et al. The quality of life of patients with end-stage renal disease. N Engl J Med. 1985;312(9):553-9.
3. Port FK, Wolfe RA, Mauger EA, et al. Comparison of survival probabilities for dialysis patients vs cadaveric renal transplant recipients. JAMA. 1993;270(11): 1339-43.
4. Organ Procurement and Transplantation Network (OPTN) and Scientific Registry of Transplant Recipients (SRTR). OPTN/SRTR 2011 Annual Data Report. Rockville, MD: Department of Health and Human Services, Health Resources and Services Administration, Healthcare Systems Bureau, Division of Transplantation; 2012:11-46.
5. Ozawa M, Terasaki PI, Castro R, et al. 14th International HLA and Immunogenetics Workshop Prospective Chronic Rejection Project: a 3-year follow-up analysis. Clin Transplant. 2007:255-60.

6. Caro-Oleas JL, Gonzalez-Escribano MF, Gonzalez-Roncero FM, et al. Clinical relevance of HLA donor-specific antibodies detected by single antigen assay in kidney transplantation. Nephrol Dial Transplant. 2012;27(3):1231-8.
7. Otten HG, Verhaar MC, Borst HP, et al. Pretransplant donor-specific HLA class-I and -II antibodies are associated with an increased risk for kidney graft failure. Am J Transplant. 2012;12(6):1618-23.
8. Fidler SJ, Irish AB, Lim W, et al. Pre-transplant donor specific anti-HLA antibody is associated with antibody-mediated rejection, progressive graft dysfunction and patient death. Transplant Immunol. 2013;28(4):148-53.
9. Wu P, Jin J, Everly MJ, et al. Impact of alloantibody strength in crossmatch negative DSA positive kidney transplantation. Clin Biochem. 2013;46(15):1389-93.
10. Mohan S, Palanisamy A, Tsapepas D, et al. Donor-specific antibodies adversely affect kidney allograft outcomes. JASN. 2012;23(12):2061-71.
11. Everly MJ, Rebellato LM, Haisch CE, et al. Incidence and impact of de novo donor-specific alloantibody in primary renal allografts. Transplantation. 2013;95(3):410-17.
12. Wiebe C, Gibson IW, Blydt-Hansen TD, et al. Evolution and clinical pathologic correlations of de novo donor-specific HLA antibody post kidney transplant. Am J Transplant. 2012;12(5):1157-67.
13. Tait BD, Hudson F, Brewin G, et al. Solid phase HLA antibody detection technology-challenges in interpretation. Tissue Antigens. 2010;76(2):87-95.
14. Honger G, Hopfer H, Arnold ML, et al. Pretransplant IgG subclasses of donor-specific human leukocyte antigen antibodies and development of antibody-mediated rejection. Transplantation. 2011;92(1):41-7.
15. Loupy A, Lefaucheur C, Vernerey D, et al. Complement-binding anti-HLA antibodies and kidney-allograft survival. N Engl J Med. 2013;369(13):1215-26.
16. Crespo M, Torio A, Mas V, et al. Clinical relevance of pretransplant anti-HLA donor-specific antibodies: does C1q-fixation matter? Transplant Immunol. 2013; 29(1-4):28-33.
17. Friedlander R, Putheti P, Diaz E, et al. On the detection of anti-HLA antibodies using single antigen bead Luminex assay: lot-to-lot variations in MFI. Transplantation. 2013;96(4):e24-6.
18. Gebel HM, Liwski RS, Bray RA. Technical aspects of HLA antibody testing. Curr Opin Organ Transplant. 2013;18(4):455-62.
19. Tait BD, Susal C, Gebel HM, et al. Consensus guidelines on the testing and clinical management issues associated with HLA and non-HLA antibodies in transplantation. Transplantation. 2013;95(1):19-47.
20. Haas M, Sis B, Racusen LC, et al. Banff 2013 meeting report: inclusion of c4d-negative antibody-mediated rejection and antibody-associated arterial lesions. Am J Transplant. 2014;14(2):272-83.
21. Solez K, Colvin RB, Racusen LC, et al. Banff 07 classification of renal allograft pathology: updates and future directions. Am J Transplant. 2008;8(4):753-60.
22. Papadimitriou JC, Drachenberg CB, Ramos E, et al. Antibody-mediated allograft rejection: morphologic spectrum and serologic correlations in surveillance and for cause biopsies. Transplantation. 2013;95(1):128-36.
23. Loupy A, Suberbielle-Boissel C, Hill GS, et al. Outcome of subclinical antibody-mediated rejection in kidney transplant recipients with preformed donor-specific antibodies. Am J Transplant. 2009;9(11):2561-70.
24. Fehr T, Gaspert A. Antibody-mediated kidney allograft rejection: therapeutic options and their experimental rationale. Transpl Int. 2012;25(6):623-32.

25. Toki D, Ishida H, Horita S, et al. Impact of low-dose rituximab on splenic B cells in ABO-incompatible renal transplant recipients. Transpl Int. 2009;22(4):447-54.
26. Perry DK, Burns JM, Pollinger HS, et al. Proteasome inhibition causes apoptosis of normal human plasma cells preventing alloantibody production. Am J Transplant. 2009;9(1):201-9.
27. Soulillou JP, Guyot C, Guimbretiere J, et al. Plasma exchange in early kidney graft rejection associated with anti-donor antibodies. Nephron. 1983;35(3):158-62.
28. Roberts DM, Jiang SH, Chadban SJ. The treatment of acute antibody-mediated rejection in kidney transplant recipients-a systematic review. Transplantation. 2012;94(8):775-83.
29. Venetz JP, Pascual M. New treatments for acute humoral rejection of kidney allografts. Expert Opin Investig Drugs. 2007;16(5):625-33.
30. Jordan SC, Tyan D, Czer L, et al. Immunomodulatory actions of intravenous immunoglobulin (IVIG): potential applications in solid organ transplant recipients. Pediatr Transplant. 1998;2(2):92-105.
31. Casadei DH, del CRM, Opelz G, et al. A randomized and prospective study comparing treatment with high-dose intravenous immunoglobulin with monoclonal antibodies for rescue of kidney grafts with steroid-resistant rejection. Transplantation. 2001;71(1):53-8.
32. Stegall MD, Gloor J, Winters JL, et al. A comparison of plasmapheresis versus high-dose IVIG desensitization in renal allograft recipients with high levels of donor specific alloantibody. Am J Transplant. 2006;6(2):346-51.
33. Kaposztas Z, Podder H, Mauiyyedi S, et al. Impact of rituximab therapy for treatment of acute humoral rejection. Clin Transplant. 2009;23(1):63-73.
34. Lefaucheur C, Nochy D, Andrade J, et al. Comparison of combination Plasmapheresis/IVIg/anti-CD20 versus high-dose IVIg in the treatment of antibody-mediated rejection. Am J Transplant. 2009;9(5):1099-107.
35. Everly MJ, Everly JJ, Susskind B, et al. Bortezomib provides effective therapy for antibody- and cell-mediated acute rejection. Transplantation. 2008;86(12):1754-61.
36. Everly MJ, Everly JJ, Arend LJ, et al. Reducing de novo donor-specific antibody levels during acute rejection diminishes renal allograft loss. Am J Transplant. 2009;9(5):1063-71.
37. Flechner SM, Fatica R, Askar M, et al. The role of proteasome inhibition with bortezomib in the treatment of antibody-mediated rejection after kidney-only or kidney-combined organ transplantation. Transplantation. 2010;90(12):1486-92.
38. Waiser J, Budde K, Schutz M, et al. Comparison between bortezomib and rituximab in the treatment of antibody-mediated renal allograft rejection. Nephrol Dial Transplant. 2012;27(3):1246-51.
39. Locke JE, Magro CM, Singer AL, et al. The use of antibody to complement protein C5 for salvage treatment of severe antibody-mediated rejection. Am J Transplant. 2009;9(1):231-5.
40. Gonzalez-Roncero F, Suner M, Bernal G, et al. Eculizumab treatment of acute antibody-mediated rejection in renal transplantation: case reports. Transplant Proc. 2012;44(9):2690-4.
41. Stegall MD, Diwan T, Raghavaiah S, et al. Terminal complement inhibition decreases antibody-mediated rejection in sensitized renal transplant recipients. Am J Transplant. 2011;11(11):2405-13.
42. Haas M. Pathologic features of antibody-mediated rejection in renal allografts: an expanding spectrum. Curr Opin Nephrol Hypertens. 2012;21(3):264-71.

43. Kraus ES, Parekh RS, Oberai P, et al. Subclinical rejection in stable positive crossmatch kidney transplant patients: incidence and correlations. Am J Transplant. 2009;9(8):1826-34.
44. Fotheringham J, Angel CA, McKane W. Transplant glomerulopathy: morphology, associations and mechanism. Nephron Clin Pract. 2009;113(1):c1-7.
45. Issa N, Cosio FG, Gloor JM, et al. Transplant glomerulopathy: risk and prognosis related to anti-human leukocyte antigen class II antibody levels. Transplantation. 2008;86(5):681-5.
46. Billing H, Rieger S, Ovens J, et al. Successful treatment of chronic antibody-mediated rejection with IVIG and rituximab in pediatric renal transplant recipients. Transplantation. 2008;86(9):1214-21.
47. Hong YA, Kim HG, Choi SR, et al. Effectiveness of rituximab and intravenous immunoglobulin therapy in renal transplant recipients with chronic active antibody-mediated rejection. Transplant Proc. 2012;44(1):182-4.
48. Ishida H, Furusawa M, Shimizu T, et al. Influence of preoperative anti-HLA antibodies on short- and long-term graft survival in recipients with or without rituximab treatment. Transplant Int. 2014;27(4):371-82.

Management of Kidney Transplant Recipients with Polyomavirus Nephropathy

CHAPTER 10

Patricia Myers-Gurevitch, Darshana M Dadhania

ABSTRACT

Replication of BK virus (BKV) in the urine and/or blood is a common occurrence in kidney transplant recipients. Detection of BKV replication is associated with an increased risk for developing nephropathy and subsequent graft loss. Management of BKV replication and nephropathy is particularly challenging since antiviral medications on the market do not effectively target BK. According to a recent registry analysis in United States, the incidence of BKV-related complications have increased and 823 grafts were lost secondary to BKV-related complications.[1] This chapter reviews the diagnosis and management of BKV nephropathy, a challenging complication post kidney transplantation.

INTRODUCTION

BK virus is a member of the Polyomavirus family, along with JCV, KI virus, WU virus, Merckel cell carcinoma virus, and Simian Virus 40 (SV40). Prior to entering the teen years, >90% of individuals have been exposed to BKV as evidenced by the presence of BKV-specific antibodies in the circulation. Initial infection is associated with mild symptoms, upper respiratory infection, or cystitis.[2] The virus has tropism for the lower and upper urinary tract, where it produces a latent infection in the renal tubular epithelial cells and urothelium of normal human host.[3] The intact immune system effectively prevents uncontrolled virus replication.

Intermittent urinary shedding of BKV occurs in 5–10% of asymptomatic immunocompetent individuals.[4] In states of altered immune function, the rate of urinary shedding can dramatically increase to 20–60%. Urinary shedding is associated with appearance of decoy cells in the urine (tubular epithelial or urothelial cells with intranuclear viral inclusions).[5] In kidney transplant recipients, BKV reactivation has been associated with hematuria, ureteral stenosis, malignancy and nephropathy.[6] BKV reactivation in kidney transplant recipients is worrisome because of its propensity to cause local damage and incite an inflammatory response resulting in acute kidney injury and possible graft loss.[7]

BKV REPLICATION

In kidney transplant recipients, BKV replication can be detected in the urine within weeks of transplantation. At our center, we measured BKV replication using BKV VP1 mRNA and found the incidence to be 10% at 1 month, 20% at 3 months, 30% at 6 months and 12 months post-transplantation.[8] These data are consistent with reports from other studies that documented viruria rates of 19–49% within the first year post-transplantation utilizing DNA based PCR assays[9,10] and 30% by urine electron microscopy (EM) to identify decoy cells.[11] Incidence of BK viremia is less common and varies from 11% to 29%.[12,13] The presence of viremia indicates a more extensive infection. Ultimately, sustained viremia is associated with BKVN in 1–8% of individuals.[14] Data from the United States suggest that the cumulative incidence of BK virus-associated nephropathy (BKVN) rose from 2% at 1 year to 3.5% at 2 years to 6.6% at 5 years post-transplantation.[1]

The main risk factor for BKV replication and hence BKVN is the relative potency of immunosuppression. Factors that have been suggested to play a role include induction with antithymocyte immunoglobulin, pulse steroid therapy, maintenance steroid therapy, and tacrolimus-based immunosuppression.[8,15] In addition, recipient humoral and cellular immunity as well as virus properties associated with virulence and immune evasion may play a role.[16,17] Other risk factors include BKV seropositive donors, ischemic injury to the graft, male gender, older age, and recipient diabetes.[18] Current data suggest that early recognition of BKV replication and modulation of immune therapy, allowing for effective immune response against the virus, results in clearance of viremia and prevention of nephropathy.[19]

BKV IN THE ALLOGRAFT

BKV infection in the allograft is patchy in nature; not all cells are infected. During states of active replication, the infection spreads from the lower urinary tract to the medulla and then finally reaches the cortex. As a result to rule in the diagnosis of BKVN, the biopsy sample must be adequate and should contain some medullary tissue.

Histology

The gold standard for diagnosis of BKVN is a transplant kidney biopsy that demonstrates the presence of ground glass intranuclear inclusions and typical virus induced cytopathic changes of the renal tubular epithelial cells. Positive immunohistochemical stain of intranuclear inclusions using an antibody targeting the large T antigen confirms the diagnosis of the BKVN.[20] Typically allograft damage associated with BKVN progresses

Table 10.1: Patterns of histological changes associated with BKVN

Stage	*A*	*B (B1, B2, B3)*	*C*
Cytopathic changes	Mild	Extensive	Variable
Inflammation (tissue involvement)	<10%	Variable (>10–25%)	Variable, chronic (<50%)
Fibrosis (tissue involvement)	<10%	<50%	>50%

Adapted from Drachenberg et al.[21]

from early lesions demonstrating normal renal parenchyma with scattered tubular epithelial cells staining positive for the large T antigen to diffuse cytopathic changes associated with positive immunohistochemical staining, inflammation, and tubular damage. Persistent infection eventually leads to interstitial fibrosis and chronic inflammation with scattered nuclei staining positive for the large T antigen.

Retrospective review of a large number of BKVN-associated biopsies performed at University of Maryland characterized the histological changes into three categories, Patterns A, B and C (Table 10.1).[21] These categories correlated with the graft outcome in this group of kidney transplant recipients. Pattern A was associated with the best prognosis, graft loss of only 15%, while Patterns B and C were associated with a much higher risk of graft loss, 50% and >80%, respectively. In the 2009 Banff criteria, there is a slight modification of these categories using the semiquantified viral load identified on biopsy specimens. According to Banff 2009, stage A is an early infection, stage B is associated with more diffuse infection and stage C is associated with late infection where there is significant scarring. BKVN diagnosis associated with minimal inflammation and minimal scarring has the best prognosis, while the majority of kidney transplant recipients with significant inflammation and/or scarring are at risk for persistent allograft dysfunction or progressive decline in kidney function.[22]

The type of cellular infiltration associated with BKVN within the transplanted kidney is very similar to that of acute rejection. Others and we have demonstrated that the mRNA transcripts that are upregulated during rejection of kidney transplants are also present at the time of BKVN diagnosis.[23,24] This poses a particular challenge in the management of kidney transplant recipients whose biopsies demonstrate significant inflammation at the time of BKVN diagnosis. The trigger for BKV replication is excess immunosuppression and therefore the management is to reduce immunosuppressive therapies. However, reduction in immunosuppressive therapies in the setting of BKVN with lot of inflammation results in uncontrolled antiallograft response (an aggressive rejection episode) that results in graft loss. Because of these devastating consequences, the current approach is to use noninvasive tools to diagnose BKV replication early, prior to the onset of florid BKVN.

Noninvasive Diagnosis

Noninvasive assays to diagnose BKV replication and BKVN are very attractive, given the patchy nature of BKV infection within the transplanted kidney. The earliest assay that was used to diagnose BKV replication relied on the detection of virus-infected cells in the urine. The cellular fraction of the urine was examined under the microscope to look for virus-infected cells exhibiting typical ground glass appearance of the nucleus resulting from intranuclear virus inclusions.[25] Evaluation of "negatively-stained" urine specimens using EM identified the typical icosahedral-shaped virions. With the advent of polymerase chain reaction (PCR), the diagnosis of BKV replication has become faster and easier. The most common method used to diagnose BKV replication is measurement of BKV DNA copy numbers using real-time quantitative PCR assay. The copies can be measured in the urine or in plasma. We have developed and validated a noninvasive assay for the diagnosis of BKV replication and BKVN using urinary cell mRNA assay. In a cohort of 89 kidney transplant recipients, our urinary cell mRNA assay was diagnostic of BKVN with 100% sensitivity and 97% specificity, giving us a positive predictive value of 86% in our study cohort.[23,26]

Recently, a group from the University of North Carolina introduced the urinary Haufen assay as an accurate predictor of BKVN. Urinary Haufen are "cast-like Polyomavirus aggregates" that are detected in the urine using EM.[27] The authors compared the diagnostic utility of current noninvasive tests in clinical practice to urinary Haufen and found that urinary Haufen was associated with the highest specificity and positive predictive value. Although not compared directly, it is important to note that urine BKV VP1 mRNA assay was also associated with similar specificity and positive predictive value.

MANAGEMENT OF BKV REPLICATION AND BKVN

The cornerstone of managing BKV replication/nephropathy is reduction in immunosuppression. In kidney transplant recipients, BKV infection progresses in stages: viruria to viruria+viremia to viruria+viremia+nephropathy to graft loss. Persistent high level of BKV replication results in progressive allograft inflammation and fibrosis. Given the high risk of early graft loss associated with BKVN, it is best to detect BKV replication early and initiate pre-emptive therapy.[19]

Pre-emptive Reduction in Immunosuppressive Therapies

In the current era, noninvasive monitoring for BKV replication has become a routine practice and most centers have developed protocols for initiating pre-emptive reduction in immunosuppressive therapies in the hopes of preventing BKVN. In a prospective study of 62 transplant kidney recipients, the incidence of viruria and viremia was 64% and 22%, respectively.[28] Of the 13 individuals with viremia, 100% had clearance of viremia by median of 2 months follow-up. Similarly in another study of 123 transplant kidney recipients, 10 of 11 with BKV viremia responded and cleared their viremia at a median of 5 months following reduction in immunosuppression.[10] In a recent prospective monitoring study of kidney transplant recipients, the authors found that 16% developed BK viremia and despite reduction in immunosuppression, 47% developed BKVN.[29] There were four graft losses among the 57 kidney transplant recipients with BK viremia. These data suggest that even with systematic monitoring for BKV viremia, a small percentage of kidney transplant recipients will present with biopsy confirmed BKVN.

A systematic three-step approach to reduction in immunosuppression was designed and evaluated by Schaub and colleagues in kidney transplant recipients with viremia, presumptive BKVN (high level viremia) and biopsy confirmed BKVN (Table 10.2). In this study, step 1 was a reduction in tacrolimus to a target trough of 6–8 ng/mL. Step 2 was further reduction in tacrolimus to 4–6 ng/mL, and step 3 was 50% reduction in MMF (mycophenolate mofetil). In this prospective study, they found step 1 cleared

Table 10.2: Stepwise reduction in immunosuppression

	BKVN (n = 13)	*Presumptive BKVN (n = 17)*	*Low level BKV viremia (n = 8)*
Diagnostic criteria	Positive histology	BKV copies >10K	BKV copies <10K
Median months post-transplant (range)	4 (1.6, 7.7)	3 (1.2, 13.1)	4.7 (1.8, 7.3)
Median creatinine (range)	1.8 (1.0, 3.6)	1.7 (0.9, 4.6)	1.3 (1.0, 3.1)
Step 1* – % cleared	15%	47%	100%
Step 1+2† – % cleared	62%	88%	–
Step 1+2+3‡ – % cleared	92%	–	–
Rejection complication (clinical and subclinical)	38%	24%	13%

Adapted from Schaub et al.[30]

*Step 1 = reduction in tacrolimus to level of 6–8 ng/mL.

†Step 2 = reduction in tacrolimus to level of 4–6 ng/mL.

‡Step 3 = 50% reduction in mycophenolate mofetil.

viremia in 100% of kidney transplant recipients (n=8) with <10,000 copies/mL of BKV, 47% (8/17) of those with presumptive BKVN (>10,000 copies/mL of BKV) and 15% (2/13) of those with BKVN. Steps 1 and 2 cleared BKV viremia in 88% (15/17) of those with presumptive BKVN and 61% (8/13) of those with BKVN. Finally, Steps 1–3 cleared BKV viremia in 92% of individuals with biopsy proven BKVN. However, they found the incidence of acute rejection (subclinical + clinical) to be 24% in those with presumptive BKVN and 38% in those with biopsy-proven BKVN.[30] These data suggest that clearance of BKV viremia is achieved easily in those with low copies of BKV. In those with presumptive BKVN, clearance of BK viremia is also possible with systematic reduction in immunosuppressive therapies, but at the expense of subclinical or clinical acute rejection. Therefore, kidney transplant recipients who develop BKV viremia must be monitored closely for signs of allograft dysfunction, not only during the viremic phase but also after clearance of viremia.

Another strategy to prevent BKVN is to combine reduction of immunosuppression with a change in the type of maintenance immunosuppressive therapy. Both cyclosporine and rapamycin have been associated with lower incidence of BKV replication.[31-33] Preliminary data suggest that initiation of rapamycin to manage BKV replication may be associated with faster clearance of BKV viremia.[34] Larger studies are necessary to clarify the role of rapamycin in the management of BKVN.

Management of Biopsy Confirmed BKVN

There are many agents that have been studied for the management of BKVN, but only reduction in immunosuppressive therapies has been shown to prevent the development of BKVN. The challenge is how much reduction and for how long. Reduction of immunosuppression in kidney transplant recipients with BKV replication/BKVN is associated with increased risk of rejection and graft loss. In a study by Vasudev and colleagues where kidney transplant recipients with BKVN were managed with reduction in immunosuppression, the 3-year actuarial graft survival rate was only 58%.[35]

The optimal management for individuals with BKVN associated with florid inflammation and tubulitis is an interesting challenge, since it is difficult to rule in or rule out the presence of concurrent rejection. In a retrospective study, the outcomes of transplant kidney recipients with BKVN who had concurrent inflammation/tubulitis were evaluated. In this study, one group had received pulse steroids initially followed by reduction in immunosuppression, the second group had received reduction in immunosuppression only, and the third group had no change in immunosuppression. In their study, reduction in immunosuppression compared to pulse steroids in conjunction with reduction of maintenance immunosuppression was associated with less cytopathic changes in the kidney.[36] Pulse steroids also resulted in improvement in tubulitis but this effect was not associated with improvement in kidney function.

Because of their in vitro antiviral properties, prophylactic fluoroquinolones have also been studied to prevent and treat BKV reactivation.[37,38] A prospective double-blinded placebo controlled trial performed in 39 transplant kidney recipients evaluated if levofloxacin therapy is associated with improved clearance of would BKV compared to placebo. In this study, the authors found no significant difference between levofloxacin therapy and placebo.[39]

Human intravenous immunoglobulin (IVIG) contains antibodies reactive against BKV and also has anti-inflammatory properties. As a result, it has been used to manage transplant kidney recipients with BKVN.[40,41] Studies indicate that treatment with IVIG in combination with reduction in immunosuppression is associated with clearance of viremia and histological improvement.[42] Recently, a case report suggested that the use of IVIG was actually associated with increase in BKV copies.[43] Since IVIG does have immunomodulatory properties, it is possible that the use of IVIG resulted in an increase in total immunosuppression in this individual and thus resulted in a rise in BKV. Prospective controlled trials are required to evaluate if the use of IVIG as an anti-inflammatory agent is useful in the management of BKVN.

At the current time, there are no antiviral drugs that have been proven to be effective in suppressing BKV replication in vivo. Centers have published their results on the use of various agents that may be useful in the management of BKVN.[44] Cidofovir, a nucleoside analogue, may affect BKV replication by interfering with large T antigen expression. It has been used for management of BKV replication in HSCT (hematopoietic stem cell transplant) recipients and in those with kidney transplants.[45] At least 184 kidney transplant recipients with BKVN have been managed with cidofovir and of those only 49% cleared their viremia.[46] Twenty-three percent experienced early graft loss. Treatment with cidofovir is limited by its potential for nephrotoxicity. Currently, a newer agent that is a lipid conjugate of cidofovir, CXM001, is being studied for management of BKV associated hemorrhagic cystitis and BKVN.[47]

In addition to antiviral/antibacterial agents, leflunomide, an anti-inflammatory agent used in patients with rheumatoid arthritis, has also been used to manage transplant kidney recipients with BKVN.[48] Metabolite(s) of leflunomide inhibit protein kinase activity and pyrimidine synthesis and can reduce BKV replication in vitro. Treatment with leflunomide has also been shown to decrease BKV replication in kidney transplant recipients.[49,50] However, there are no randomized controlled trials demonstrating its effectiveness, and it has been associated with significant liver toxicity and hemolysis. FK778 is a drug that is closely related to the active metabolite of leflunomide. A phase 2 randomized controlled trial that compared MMF or FK778 based maintenance immunosuppression did not demonstrate a benefit in preventing BK viruria or viremia.[51]

At out center we have utilized a combination of IVIG, reduction in immunosuppressive medications and conversion of mycophenolate mofetil to leflunomide.[52] Our data suggest that 66% have complete clearance of viremia by the end of 6 months and the risk of graft loss is significantly decreased compared to the historical control that did not receive this combination of therapies.

When the patient presents with BKVN, one is obligated to intervene to avoid progression to graft loss and the intervention that is common to all protocols is reduction in immunosuppression. Johnston and colleagues pooled all the existing data on three different strategies to manage BKVN—reduction in immunosuppressive therapies (IS) alone vs cidofovir plus reduction in IS vs leflunomide with reduction in IS.[53] The graft failure rate was not significantly different between the three groups. As a result they concluded that there is no convincing evidence that the use of adjuvant therapies provides additional benefit to reduction in IS alone for management of BKVN kidney transplant recipients. Overall reduction in immunosuppression has resulted in resolution of BKVN and lower rates of graft loss with improved overall graft survival.[22] However, >30–50% of individuals continue to have significant decrease in kidney function following BKVN diagnosis.[54]

Retransplantation Following Allograft Loss Due to BKVN

Risk of graft loss and persistent graft dysfunction following BKVN diagnosis is high. Having suffered a graft loss, many of these transplant kidney recipients return to the waiting list.[55] Although these patients tend to be more sensitized, graft loss due to BKVN is not a contraindication to retransplantation. The most important factor in preventing BKVN in the subsequent graft is clearance of BKV viremia/viruria prior to retransplantation.[56] Furthermore, at this time there are no recommendations for avoiding any specific immunosuppressive therapy at the time of subsequent transplant. Most recipients with failed graft due to BKVN have been transplanted with their centers' standard immunosuppressive protocols.

BKV AND MALIGNANCY

In the current literature, BKV has also been associated with malignancy. In our institution, we encountered a case of microinvasive urothelial carcinoma localized to the transplant kidney 7 years following the diagnosis of BKVN.[57] Our patient had resolution of both BKV viremia and BKV associated

Table 10.3: Proposed mechanisms of BKV associated oncogenesis

Virus protein	*Proposed mechanism*
Large T antigen	Binds and blocks tumor suppressor proteins (p53 and pRB family of proteins
Large T antigen	Causes structural chromosomal alterations by binding to topoisomerase I
Large T antigen	Causes structural chromosomal alterations via its helicase activity
Small t antigen	Inactivates the function of PP2A (a protein phosphatase that has tumor suppressor activity)

Adapted from Tognon et al.[58]

histological changes within 1 year following BKV diagnosis. However, the tumor cells stained diffusely positive for BKV.

Evidence suggesting that the BKV can play a role in the induction and progression of human tumors is summarized in Table 10.3 and includes the following: (1) BKV does produce a latent infection, (2) the expression of large T and small t antigens can disrupt normal cell growth by interfering with tumor suppressor genes, and (3) BKV can cause structural alterations in the host DNA. In addition to uncontrolled virus replication during an immunosuppressed state, there may be uncoupling of capsid protein expression, viron assembly, and cell lysis that drives the development of malignancy.[58]

Although BKV has been suggested to be the driver in the development of malignancy, there are other possible explanations for the observed association between BKV and malignancy. A "hit and run" hypothesis suggests that BKV infection causes chromosomal instability that promotes malignant transformation even after BKV infection has resolved. The "passenger" role would be evoked if BKV finds favorable conditions for replication in an already transformed cell, and BKV is not directly contributing to the oncogenic properties of that cell. Lastly, the "by-stander" role would suggest that BKV infects neighboring cells, or is detectable in body compartments that are nearby but is not directly related to the development of the malignancy. The WHO International Agency for Cancer Research Monograph Working Group has classified BKV as "possible carcinogenic to humans".[44]

SUMMARY

BKV reactivation post kidney transplantation is common and is associated with increased risk of graft dysfunction. The lack of effective antiviral therapy for BKV results in a challenging management problem for transplant physicians. At this time, data suggest that prevention of BKVN through prospective monitoring and pre-emptive reduction in immunosuppression is a reasonable approach. Persistent viremia should lead to a kidney biopsy to assess the histological stage of BKVN and to determine prognosis. The risk of graft loss remains high in individuals with BKVN and concurrent inflammation. Randomized controlled trials to evaluate novel therapies and their potential advantage over reduction in immunosuppressive therapies alone are needed. In addition, development and validation of noninvasive biomarkers to monitor BKV replication and associated inflammatory response are necessary to enhance the management of transplant kidney recipients with BKVN.

REFERENCES

1. Dharnidharka VR, Cherikh WS, Abbott KC. An OPTN analysis of national registry data on treatment of BK virus allograft nephropathy in the United States. Transplantation 2009;87(7):1019-26.
2. Knowles WA, Pipkin P, Andrews N, et al. Population-based study of antibody to the human polyomaviruses BKV and JCV and the simian polyomavirus SV40. J Med Virol. 2003;71(1):115-23.
3. Imperiale MJ. The human polyomaviruses, BKV and JCV: molecular pathogenesis of acute disease and potential role in cancer. Virology. 2000;267(1):1-7.
4. Markowitz RB, Thompson HC, Mueller JF, et al. Incidence of BK virus and JC virus viruria in human immunodeficiency virus-infected and -uninfected subjects. J Infect Dis. 1993;167(1):13-20.
5. Singh HK, Bubendorf L, Mihatsch MJ, et al. Urine cytology findings of polyomavirus infections. Adv Exp Med Biol. 2006;577:201-12.
6. Randhawa P, Brennan DC. BK virus infection in transplant recipients: an overview and update. Am J Transplant. 2006;6(9):2000-5.
7. Purighalla R, Shapiro R, McCauley J, et al. BK virus infection in a kidney allograft diagnosed by needle biopsy. Am J Kidney Dis. 1995;26(4):671-3.
8. Dadhania D, Snopkowski C, Ding R, et al. Epidemiology of BK virus in renal allograft recipients: independent risk factors for BK virus replication. Transplantation. 2008;86(4):521-8.
9. Babel N, Fendt J, Karaivanov S, et al. Sustained BK viruria as an early marker for the development of BKV-associated nephropathy: analysis of 4128 urine and serum samples. Transplantation. 2009;88(1):89-95.
10. Almeras C, Foulongne V, Garrigue V, et al. Does reduction in immunosuppression in viremic patients prevent BK virus nephropathy in de novo renal transplant recipients? A prospective study. Transplantation. 2008;85(8):1099-104.
11. Hirsch HH, Knowles W, Dickenmann M, et al. Prospective study of polyomavirus type BK replication and nephropathy in renal-transplant recipients. N Engl J Med. 2002;347(7):488-96.
12. Agha I, Brennan DC. BK virus and immunosuppressive agents. Adv Exp Med Biol. 2006;577:174-84.
13. Bressollette-Bodin C, Coste-Burel M, Hourmant M, et al. A prospective longitudinal study of BK virus infection in 104 renal transplant recipients. Am J Transplant. 2005;5(8):1926-33.

14. Hirsch HH, Brennan DC, Drachenberg CB, et al. Polyomavirus-associated nephropathy in renal transplantation: interdisciplinary analyses and recommendations. Transplantation. 2005;79(10):1277-86.
15. Acott P, Babel N. BK virus replication following kidney transplant: does the choice of immunosuppressive regimen influence outcomes? Ann Transplant. 2012;17(1):86-99.
16. Babel N, Volk HD, Reinke P. BK polyomavirus infection and nephropathy: the virus-immune system interplay. Nat Rev Nephrol. 2011;7(7):399-406.
17. Medeiros M, Dadhania D, Velásquez-Jones L Nefropatía por virus BK. In: Alberú J, Morales JL (Eds.). Infecciones en el paciente receptor de trasplante renal. Barcelona: Publicaciones Permanyer; 2012;123-127.
18. Hirsch HH, Drachenberg CB, Steiger J, et al. Polyomavirus-associated nephropathy in renal transplantation: critical issues of screening and management. Adv Exp Med Biol. 2006;577:160-73.
19. Ramos E, Drachenberg CB, Wali R, et al. The decade of polyomavirus BK-associated nephropathy: state of affairs. Transplantation. 2009;87(5):621-30.
20. Drachenberg CB, Hirsch HH, Ramos E, et al. Polyomavirus disease in renal transplantation: review of pathological findings and diagnostic methods. Hum Pathology. 2005;36(12):1245-55.
21. Drachenberg CB, Papadimitriou JC, Hirsch HH, et al. Histological patterns of polyomavirus nephropathy: correlation with graft outcome and viral load. Am J Transplant. 2004;4(12):2082-92.
22. Masutani K, Shapiro R, Basu A, et al. The Banff 2009 Working Proposal for polyomavirus nephropathy: a critical evaluation of its utility as a determinant of clinical outcome. Am J Transplant. 2012;12(4):907-18.
23. Dadhania D, Snopkowski C, Ding R, et al. Validation of noninvasive diagnosis of BK virus nephropathy and identification of prognostic biomarkers. Transplantation. 2010;90(2):189-97.
24. Mannon RB, Hoffmann SC, Kampen RL, et al. Molecular evaluation of BK polyomavirus nephropathy. Am J Transplant. 2005;5(12):2883-93.
25. Nickeleit V, Klimkait T, Binet IF, et al. Testing for polyomavirus type BK DNA in plasma to identify renal-allograft recipients with viral nephropathy. N Engl J Med. 2000;342(18):1309-15.
26. Ding R, Medeiros M, Dadhania D, et al. Noninvasive diagnosis of BK virus nephritis by measurement of messenger RNA for BK virus VP1 in urine. Transplantation. 2002;74(7):987-94.
27. Singh HK, Andreoni KA, Madden V, et al. Presence of urinary Haufen accurately predicts polyomavirus nephropathy. JASN. 2009;20(2):416-27.
28. Ginevri F, Azzi A, Hirsch HH, et al. Prospective monitoring of polyomavirus BK replication and impact of pre-emptive intervention in pediatric kidney recipients. Am J Transplant. 2007;7(12):2727-35.
29. Knight RJ, Gaber LW, Patel SJ, et al. Screening for BK viremia reduces but does not eliminate the risk of BK nephropathy. Transplantation. 2013;96(7):e51.
30. Schaub S, Hirsch HH, Dickenmann M, et al. Reducing immunosuppression preserves allograft function in presumptive and definitive polyomavirus-associated nephropathy. Am J Transplant. 2010;10(12):2615-23.
31. Benavides CA, Pollard VB, Mauiyyedi S, et al. BK virus-associated nephropathy in sirolimus-treated renal transplant patients: incidence, course, and clinical outcomes. Transplantation. 2007;84(1):83-8.

32. Brennan DC, Agha I, Bohl DL, et al. Incidence of BK with tacrolimus versus cyclosporine and impact of preemptive immunosuppression reduction. Am J Transplant. 2005;5(3):582-94.
33. Hirsch HH, Vincenti F, Friman S, et al. Polyomavirus BK replication in de novo kidney transplant patients receiving tacrolimus or cyclosporine: a prospective, randomized, multicenter study. Am J Transplant. 2013;13(1):136-45.
34. Sanchez Fructuoso AI, Calvo N, Perez-Flores I, et al. Mammalian target of rapamycin signal inhibitors could play a role in the treatment of BK polyomavirus nephritis in renal allograft recipients. Transpl Infect Dis. 2011;13(6):584-91.
35. Vasudev B, Hariharan S, Hussain SA, et al. BK virus nephritis: risk factors, timing, and outcome in renal transplant recipients. Kidney Int. 2005;68(4):1834-9.
36. Celik B, Shapiro R, Vats A, et al. Polyomavirus allograft nephropathy: sequential assessment of histologic viral load, tubulitis, and graft function following changes in immunosuppression. Am J Transplant. 2003;3(11):1378-82.
37. Wojciechowski D, Chanda R, Chandran S, et al. Ciprofloxacin prophylaxis in kidney transplant recipients reduces BK virus infection at 3 months but not at 1 year. Transplantation. 2012;94(11):1117-23.
38. Leung AY, Chan MT, Yuen KY, et al. Ciprofloxacin decreased polyoma BK virus load in patients who underwent allogeneic hematopoietic stem cell transplantation. Clin Infect Dis. 2005;40(4):528-37.
39. Chung BH, Hong YA, Kim HG, et al. Clinical usefulness of BK virus plasma quantitative PCR to prevent BK virus associated nephropathy. Transplant Int. 2012;25(6):687-95.
40. Sener A, House AA, Jevnikar AM, et al. Intravenous immunoglobulin as a treatment for BK virus associated nephropathy: one-year follow-up of renal allograft recipients. Transplantation. 2006;81(1):117-20.
41. Sbrana S, Ruocco L, Vanacore R, et al. In vitro effects of an immunoglobulin preparation for intravenous use (IVIG) on T-cells activation. Allerg Immunol. 1993;25(1):35-7.
42. Anyaegbu EI, Almond PS, Milligan T, et al. Intravenous immunoglobulin therapy in the treatment of BK viremia and nephropathy in pediatric renal transplant recipients. Pediatr Transplant. 2012;16(1):E19-24.
43. Maggiore U, Medici MC, Vaglio A, et al. Increased viral load after intravenous immunoglobulin therapy for BK virus-associated nephropathy. Transpl Infect Dis. 2010;12(5):470-2.
44. Dalianis T, Hirsch HH. Human polyomaviruses in disease and cancer. Virology. 2013;437(2):63-72.
45. Vats A, Shapiro R, Singh Randhawa P, et al. Quantitative viral load monitoring and cidofovir therapy for the management of BK virus-associated nephropathy in children and adults. Transplantation. 2003;75(1):105-12.
46. Hilton R, Tong CY. Antiviral therapy for polyomavirus-associated nephropathy after renal transplantation. J Antimicrob Chemother. 2008;62(5):855-9.
47. Gosert R, Rinaldo CH, Wernli M, et al. CMX001 (1-O-hexadecyloxypropyl-cidofovir) inhibits polyomavirus JC replication in human brain progenitor-derived astrocytes. Antimicrob Agents Chemother. 2011;55(5):2129-36.
48. Josephson MA, Gillen D, Javaid B, et al. Treatment of renal allograft polyoma BK virus infection with leflunomide. Transplantation. 2006;81(5):704-10.
49. Faguer S, Hirsch HH, Kamar N, et al. Leflunomide treatment for polyomavirus BK-associated nephropathy after kidney transplantation. Transplant Int. 2007;20(11):962-9.

50. Leca N. Leflunomide use in renal transplantation. Curr Opin Organ Transplant. 2009;14(4):370-4.
51. Guasch A, Roy-Chaudhury P, Woodle ES, et al. Assessment of efficacy and safety of FK778 in comparison with standard care in renal transplant recipients with untreated BK nephropathy. Transplantation. 2010;90(8):891-7.
52. Dadhania D AM, Thomas D, Lee J, et al. A pilot trial of IVIG, leflunomide and low dose tacrolimus in renal allograft recipients with BK virus nephritis. JASN 2007;18:442A.
53. Johnston O, Jaswal D, Gill JS, et al. Treatment of polyomavirus infection in kidney transplant recipients: a systematic review. Transplantation. 2010;89(9):1057-70.
54. Wadei HM, Rule AD, Lewin M, et al. Kidney transplant function and histological clearance of virus following diagnosis of polyomavirus-associated nephropathy (PVAN). Am J Transplant. 2006;6(5 Pt 1):1025-32.
55. Dharnidharka VR, Cherikh WS, Neff R, et al. Retransplantation after BK virus nephropathy in prior kidney transplant: an OPTN database analysis. Am J Transplant. 2010;10(5):1312-5.
56. Geetha D, Sozio SM, Ghanta M, et al. Results of repeat renal transplantation after graft loss from BK virus nephropathy. Transplantation. 2011;92(7):781-6.
57. Myers-Gurevitch P DD, Salvatore S, Lee JB, et al. Intrarenal urothelial carcinoma staining positive for BKV years after resolution of BKV nephropathy. JASN. 2013;24:622A.
58. Tognon M, Corallini A, Martini F, et al. Oncogenic transformation by BK virus and association with human tumors. Oncogene. 2003;22(33):5192-200.

Personalizing Immunosuppression Regimens for Kidney Transplant Recipients

CHAPTER

11

Jennifer McDermott

ABSTRACT

Kidney transplantation and associated immunosuppressive therapy have greatly evolved over the past 60 years. Several immunosuppressant medications have been approved by the FDA and used in various combinations in kidney transplantation. Both induction and maintenance immunosuppressive strategies have changed over time, resulting in lower acute allograft rejection rates and improved survival. Desensitization protocols have been developed to allow greater access to transplant for those at a higher immunological risk and human leukocyte antigen (HLA) incompatible with their donor. Despite many advances, long-term allograft survival has largely remained unchanged over the past 15 years and chronic allograft dysfunction continues to be a leading cause of graft loss. New and emerging maintenance immunosuppressive therapies have been developed that are void of nephrotoxic effects yet adequately suppress T- and B-cell pathways. Drug development and investigation has also focused on B-cell-directed therapies. Advances in immune therapy for kidney transplantation including evolution of induction and maintenance immunosuppressive regimens, desensitization protocols, and emerging therapies are reviewed in this chapter.

INTRODUCTION

Kidney transplantation and associated immunosuppressive therapy have greatly evolved over time. From the 1960s to 1970s, maintenance immunosuppressive regimens mainly consisted of two agents: corticosteroids and azathioprine. Since that time, an increasing number of maintenance immunosuppressive agents have become available for use in various combinations allowing for more choice and personalization of immunosuppressive therapy (Table 11.1). In addition, the use of specialized induction agents has increased both to prevent early acute rejection and to minimize maintenance immunosuppression (Fig. 11.1 and Table 11.1).

Despite several advancements, there are pros and cons to each immunosuppressive agent. An ideal regimen that leads to prolonged allograft and

Table 11.1: Immunosuppressive agents

Immunosuppressive agent	*Class*	*Uses in kidney transplantation*	*Adverse effects*	*Monitoring parameters*	*Additional considerations*
Antithymocyte globulin, rabbit (Thymoglobulin)	Polyclonal antibody; polyclonal IgG against human T lymphocytes derived from rabbits; reduces the number of circulating T lymphocytes, which alters T-cell activation, homing, and cytotoxic function	Induction, treatment of rejection	Leukopenia, thrombocytopenia, fever, chills, dyspnea, pulmonary edema, tachycardia, hypotension, phlebitis, pruritus, erythema, rash, serum sickness, infection	Vital signs, CBC, absolute lymphocyte count	Premedication recommended with diphenhydramine and acetaminophen
Antithymocyte globulin, equine (ATGAM)	Polyclonal antibody; polyclonal IgG against human T lymphocytes derived from horses; reduces the number of circulating T lymphocytes, which alters T-cell activation, homing, and cytotoxic function	Induction, treatment of rejection			Premedication recommended with diphenhydramine and acetaminophen test dose required (intra-dermal injection of 0.1 mL of a 1:1,000 dilution) due to risk of anaphylaxis
Basiliximab (Simulect)	Anti-CD25 monoclonal antibody; binds to the α subunit of the IL-2 receptor present only on activated and nonresting T cells	Induction	Rare; possible hypersensitivity reaction	None	
Alemtuzumab (Campath)	Anti-CD52 monoclonal antibody; binds CD52 antigen on T and B cells, NK cells, and less densely on monocytes and macrophages causing cell lysis through antibody-dependent cellular cytotoxicity resulting in profound depletion of T cells and to a lesser degree B cells and monocytes	Induction (off-label), treatment of rejection (off-label)	Leukopenia, thrombocytopenia, headache, fever, chills, dyspnea, tachycardia, hypotension, phlebitis, pruritus, erythema, rash, infection	Vital signs, CBC, absolute lymphocyte count	Premedication recommended with diphenhydramine and acetaminophen

Contd...

Contd...

Immunosuppressive agent	*Class*	*Uses in kidney transplantation*	*Adverse effects*	*Monitoring parameters*	*Additional considerations*
Corticosteroids: prednisone, prednisolone, methylprednisolone, dexamethasone	Inhibit NF-AT thereby blocking transcription of cytokine genes (interleukins 1, 2, 3, 5, TNF-alpha, and interferon gamma) and inhibiting cytokine production by T cells and macrophages	Induction, treatment of rejection, maintenance	Hyperglycemia, hypertension, hyperlipidemia, psychosis, mood swings, insomnia, photosensitivity, acne, osteoporosis, bone fractures, avascular necrosis, weight gain, fluid retention, increased appetite, hirsutism, Cushing's syndrome, menstrual irregularities, growth retardation, GI disturbance, cataracts, impaired wound healing, infection	Glucose, blood pressure, lipid panel	
Tacrolimus (Prograf and Astagraf)	Calcineurin inhibitor; results in blockade of signal transduction by NF-AT, thereby preventing gene transcription for formation of lymphokines and ultimately inhibiting T-cell activation	Maintenance	Nephrotoxicity, neurotoxicity (Tac>CsA), hyperglycemia (Tac>CsA), hypertension (CsA>Tac) hyperlipidemia (CsA>Tac), hyperkalemia, hypomagnesemia hyperuricemia, HUS/TMA, infection, gingival hyperplasia (CsA only), hirsutism (CsA only), alopecia (Tac only)	12-h trough levels (Prograf) or 24-h trough levels (Astagraf), serum creatinine, potassium, magnesium, uric acid	
Cyclosporine (Neoral, Gengraf, and Sandimmune)	Calcineurin inhibitor; results in blockade of signal transduction by NF-AT, thereby preventing gene transcription for formation of lymphokines and ultimately inhibiting T-cell activation	Maintenance		12-h trough levels or 2-h post-dose levels, serum creatinine, potassium, magnesium, uric acid	Modified formulations (Neoral and Gengraf) are not bioequivalent to nonmodified formulations (Sandimmune)
Mycophenolate mofetil (Cellcept)	Antimetabolite; inhibits lymphocyte purine synthesis by reversibly and noncompetitively inhibiting IMPDH	Maintenance	Nausea, vomiting, diarrhea, abdominal pain, leukopenia, thrombocytopenia, anemia, infection	CBC	Prodrug of mycophenolic acid
Mycophenolate sodium (Myfortic)					Delayed-release tablet of mycophenolic acid

Contd...

Contd...

mmunosuppressive agent	*Class*	*Uses in kidney transplantation*	*Adverse effects*	*Monitoring parameters*	*Additional considerations*
Azathioprine (Imuran)	Antimetabolite; metabolized to 6-mercaptopurine which is incorporated into nucleic acids (substitutes for the purine base guanine) ultimately inhibiting DNA and RNA synthesis	Maintenance	Leukopenia, thrombocytopenia, macrocytic anemia, nausea, vomiting, abdominal pain, alopecia, pancreatitis, hepatotoxicity, infection	CBC, LFT	
Sirolimus (Rapamune)	m-TOR inhibitor; blocks signal transduction pathways ultimately inhibiting IL-2 and other cytokine induced activation and proliferation of T and B cells	Maintenance	Thrombocytopenia, leukopenia, anemia, hyperlipidemia, impaired wound healing, wound-related reactions, peripheral edema, mouth ulcers, bone pain, diarrhea, proteinuria, pneumonitis, hepatic artery thrombosis in liver transplant, HUS/TMA, infection	24-h trough levels (C0), lipid panel, CBC, LFT	Frequent dosage adjustments based on nonsteady state sirolimus concentrations can lead to overdosing or underdosing due to the long elimination half-life of sirolimus
Everolimus (Zortress)	m-TOR inhibitor; blocks signal transduction pathways ultimately inhibiting IL-2 and other cytokine induced activation and proliferation of T and B cells	Maintenance	Anemia, hyperlipidemia, impaired wound healing, wound-related reactions, peripheral edema, mouth ulcers, diarrhea, proteinuria, pneumonitis, kidney graft thrombosis, hepatic artery thrombosis in liver transplant, HUS/TMA, infection	12-h trough levels (C0), lipid panel, CBC, LFT	
Belatacept (Nulojix)	Costimulation blocker; blocks the CD28 mediated costimulation of T lymphocytes by binding to CD80 and CD86 on antigen-presenting cells	Maintenance	Fever, hypertension, headache, cough, anemia, leukopenia, nausea, vomiting, diarrhea, constipation, peripheral edema, PTLD, PML, infection	EBV serostatus (prior to treatment), REMS preinfusion check list	REMS requirements to communicate the increased risk of PTLD and PML. Contraindicated in transplant recipients who are EBV seronegative or with unknown EBV serostatus

(CBC: Complete blood count; LFT: Liver function tests; NF-AT: Nuclear factor of activated T-cells; IMPDH: Inosine monophosphate dehydrogenase; m-TOR: Mammalian target of rapamycin; CsA: Cyclosporine; Tac: Tacrolimus; HUS/TMA: Hemolytic uremic syndrome/thrombotic microangiopathy; PTLD: Post-transplant lymphoproliferative disorder; PML: Progressive multifocal leukoencephalopathy; EBV: Epstein-Barr virus; REMS: Risk evaluation and mitigation strategy).

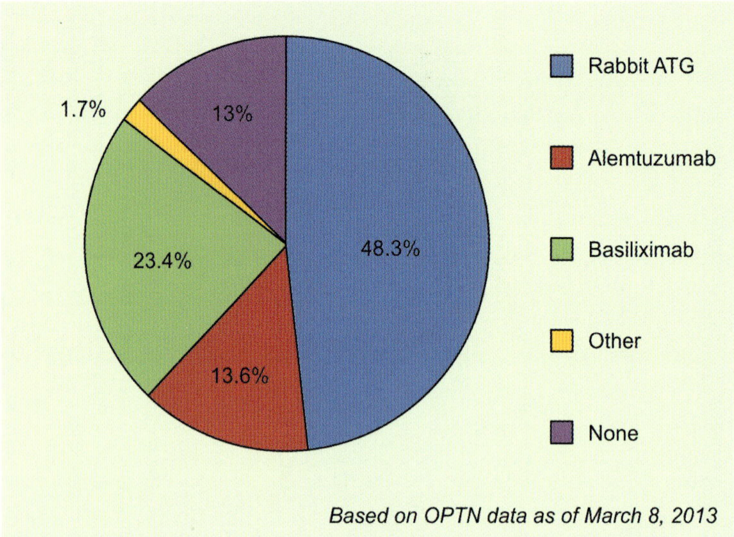

Fig. 11.1: Induction therapy for adult kidney transplant recipients in 2012.

patient survival but is void of associated morbidity including infection, malignancy, and drug-related toxicities has not yet been identified. Furthermore, long-term kidney allograft survival has only seen small improvements since 1995,[1] and death with a functioning graft, most commonly due to cardiovascular disease, is one of the leading causes of late allograft loss.[2,3] Calcineurin inhibitors, first cyclosporine and later tacrolimus, greatly reduced rejection rates and improved overall graft survival, but paradoxically are associated with significant adverse effects including nephrotoxicity, hypertension, glucose intolerance, and hyperlipidemia that can negatively impact both graft and patient survival.[4-6] While the majority of kidney transplant recipients continue to be maintained on a calcineurin inhibitor as part of their immunosuppressive regimen, several trials have been conducted aiming to avoid, minimize, withdraw, or convert calcineurin inhibitors, given their adverse effect profiles.

Corticosteroids have been a cornerstone of immunosuppressive therapy in solid organ transplantation since the 1960s and continue to be utilized as part of the maintenance immunosuppressive regimen in two-thirds of kidney transplant recipients,[7] but because they also have multiple side effects including hypertension, glucose intolerance, hyperlipidemia, and weight gain that can contribute to associated cardiovascular morbidity and mortality, strategies have been employed to minimize their use.

While these strategies may be of benefit, a one size fits all approach may not be best suited to the individual patient. When designing an immunosuppressive regimen, recipient factors including age, race, comorbidities, immunologic risk, genetic polymorphisms, concomitant and previous

Table 11.2: Select cytochrome P450 3A interactions that affect tacrolimus, cyclosporine, sirolimus and everolimus*

CYP 450 3A inhibitors	*CYP 450 3A inducers*
• Clotrimazole, fluconazole, ketoconazole, itraconazole, posaconazole, voriconazole	• Phenytoin, carbamazepine, oxcarbazepine, phenobarbital
• Erythromycin, clarithromycin, telithromycin	• Rifampin, rifabutin
• Diltiazem, verapamil	• Modafinil
• Ritonavir, saquinavir, indinavir, nelfinavir, amprenavir, lopinavir, atazanavir, fosamprenavir, tipranavir, darunavir	• Efavirenz, nevirapine, etravirine
• Telaprevir, boceprevir	• Nafcillin
• Conivaptan	• St. John's wort
• Nefazodone	
• Aprepitant	
• Isoniazid	
• Amiodarone	
• Cimetidine	
• Grapefruit, star fruit, pomegranate, ginkgo biloba	

*Note that this is not an exhaustive list.

pharmacotherapy, and overall immunosuppression burden should be considered. There are several significant drug-drug interactions with select immunosuppressive agents utilized in kidney transplant pharmacotherapy that must be considered when choosing and devising a dosing strategy for an individual immunosuppressive agent (Table 11.2). Herein, this chapter reviews considerations and supporting data for immunosuppressive agent selection and dosing when designing a regimen for the individual patient.

INDUCTION IMMUNOSUPPRESSIVE AGENT SELECTION

Induction immunosuppression is intense prophylactic therapy utilized at the time of the transplant to prevent early acute rejection. It generally consists of high-dose corticosteroids and/or other maintenance immunosuppressive agents in combination with a potent specialized agent given in the immediate perioperative period. The use of specialized induction agents has increased over time with 87% of patients undergoing kidney transplantation in the Unites States in 2012 receiving such medications based on Organ Procurement and Transplantation Network (OPTN) data. Two T-cell-depleting agents, rabbit antithymocyte (rabbit ATG, Thymoglobulin) and alemtuzumab (Campath), and one nondepleting agent, basiliximab (Simulect), compose the majority of induction use (Fig. 11.1).

While there are two ATG preparations available for use, one horse-derived product (equine ATG, ATGAM®) and one rabbit-derived product (rabbit ATG), equine ATG use fell out of favor since rabbit ATG has been associated with significantly less acute rejection, greater event-free survival, defined as freedom from death, graft loss, or rejection, and less cytomegalovirus disease.[8] These agents are prepared by immunizing horses or rabbits with human thymocytes with resulting equine or rabbit immune globulins against human T cells that are then collected and purified. ATG reduces the number of circulating T lymphocytes, which alters T-cell activation, homing, and cytotoxic function and ultimately affects cell-mediated and humoral immunity. Rabbit-derived ATG includes antibodies against several T-cell markers including CD2, CD3, CD4, CD8, CD11a, CD18, CD25, CD44, CD45, HLA-DR, HLA Class I heavy chains and beta-2 microglobulin with associated lymphocyte depletion occurring through Fc-dependent opsonization.[9–11] Common adverse effects of rabbit ATG include myelosuppression (leukopenia and thrombocytopenia), infusion-related reactions due to cytokine release, hypotension, tachycardia, and dyspnea (Table 11.1). Because of the associated infusion-related reactions, rabbit ATG requires premedication with diphenhydramine, acetaminophen, and +/− corticosteroid, a prolonged infusion rate over at least 4–6 h, careful vital sign monitoring, and rate titration. Infusion-related reactions are most pronounced during the first one to two doses. Of note, patients with cardiovascular and/or pulmonary disease should be closely monitored, given this adverse effect profile. Rabbit ATG induction dosing regimens are variable but commonly consist of 1.5 mg/kg/dose administered daily and continued for 4–5 days.

Basiliximab (Simulect), a nondepleting monoclonal antibody directed against CD25, the interleukin-2 receptor alpha chain of activated T cells, is another commonly used agent for induction therapy in kidney transplantation.[12] It is given as a fixed two-dose regimen; 20 mg intravenously on the day of the transplant and day 4 after transplantation. Advantages are that it is well tolerated and can be administered over 30 min. In placebo-controlled trials, basiliximab resulted in significantly less acute rejection but a similar incidence of adverse events and infections.[13,14] In multicenter randomized trials of adult kidney transplant recipients receiving cyclosporine, mycophenolate mofetil, corticosteroids and either rabbit ATG or basiliximab, 1 year graft survival was similar but rabbit ATG resulted in a significantly lower incidence of acute rejection, 15.6% vs 25.5%; p=0.02.[15,16] However, a greater incidence of infection (85.8% vs 75.2%; p=0.03) and leukopenia was observed with rabbit ATG (33.3% vs 14.6%; p<0.001).[15,16]

The most recent agent utilized for induction immunosuppression, due to powerful lymphocyte depleting effects, is alemtuzumab; a humanized monoclonal antibody targeting the CD52 antigen located on T and B cells, NK cells, and to a lesser degree monocytes and macrophages.[17,18]

Associated antibody-dependent cellular cytotoxicity results in profound depletion of T cells and to a lesser degree B cells and monocytes. Common adverse effects of alemtuzumab include myelosuppression (leukopenia and thrombocytopenia) as well as infusion-related reactions due to cytokine release. In the kidney transplant population, the associated infusion-related reactions tend not to be as severe as can be seen with rabbit ATG, although premedication with diphenhydramine, acetaminophen +/− corticosteroid and careful vital sign monitoring are recommended. Alemtuzumab is easily administered often given as a single 30 mg intravenous dose intraoperatively infused over 2 h. Effective September 4, 2012, alemtuzumab is no longer commercially available; rather it must be provided through the Campath Distribution Program free of charge. In order to receive Campath, the health care provider is required to document and comply with certain requirements specified by the manufacturer.[19] Alemtuzumab induction has been utilized with various maintenance immunosuppression minimization strategies.[20-23] In the INTAC trial, high immunological risk patients [repeat transplant, a peak or current value of panel-reactive antibodies (PRA) of ≥20%, or black race] were randomized to receive alemtuzumab 30 mg intravenously as a single dose on the day of transplantation or rabbit ATG 1.5 mg/kg/dose intravenously for four doses, and low immunological risk patients to receive alemtuzumab 30 mg intravenously as a single dose or basiliximab 20 mg intravenously given the day of the transplant and a second dose given on day 3, 4, or 5 after transplantation. Maintenance immunosuppression consisted of tacrolimus and mycophenolate mofetil under early corticosteroid withdrawal (CSWD). At 3 years, the rate of biopsy confirmed acute rejection in low-risk patients was lower with alemtuzumab than with basiliximab (10% vs 22%; p=0.003), but among high-risk patients, no significant difference was observed between alemtuzumab and rabbit ATG (18% vs 15%; p=0.63). Although adverse event rates were similar among treatment groups, the rate of all infectious adverse events was higher with rabbit ATG than with alemtuzumab (81% vs 60%; p=0.009) and among low-risk patients, the rate of infectious adverse events that were serious was lower with basiliximab than with alemtuzumab (22% vs 35%; p=0.02). Three-year graft survival and patient survival did not significantly differ between treatment groups.[24]

In addition to infection, there is concern of post-transplant lymphoproliferative disorder (PTLD) risk, a virally driven malignancy, with potent T-cell-depleting agents such as rabbit ATG and alemtuzumab. However, in one study, while rabbit ATG was associated with significantly increased PTLD risk (p=0.0025), alemtuzumab, basiliximab, and daclizumab were not. The authors concluded that maintenance drug selection or possibly the balance between B- and T-cell depletion may be more relevant to determine risk of PTLD.[25]

Overall, when selecting an induction immunosuppressive agent, one must carefully consider several factors including immunological risk of the patient, cumulative immunosuppression burden, concomitant maintenance immunosuppression as well as additional patient factors including age and comorbidities such as cardiovascular disease, pulmonary disease, and prior malignancy. T-cell-depleting agents such as rabbit ATG or alemtuzumab are associated with lower acute rejection rates but higher rates of leukopenia and infection as compared to basiliximab. The individual patient's risk of rejection should be carefully weighed against potential complications due to over-immunosuppression and/or drug-related toxicities.

MAINTENANCE IMMUNOSUPPRESSIVE REGIMEN SELECTION

From the 1960s to 1970s, maintenance immunosuppressive regimens mainly consisted of corticosteroids and azathioprine. Since their introduction, calcineurin inhibitors, first cyclosporine in 1983 and later tacrolimus in 1994 as part of multidrug immunosuppressive maintenance regimens, changed practice greatly resulting in reduced acute allograft rejection rates and increased allograft survival, although patterns of use for these agents have changed over time. In 1998, 67.3% of kidney transplant patients were maintained on cyclosporine vs 26.1% on tacrolimus, however by 2011; only 3.9% of patients were on cyclosporine vs 89.7% on tacrolimus.[7] This trend is likely attributed to the significantly lower incidence of acute rejection observed with tacrolimus based therapy.[26-28] Despite this, cyclosporine remains an alternative agent in patients that do not tolerate tacrolimus with conversion demonstrated to be potentially useful in patients with severe neurotoxicity (i.e. seizures and mental status changes) and in management of new onset diabetes after transplant.[29,30] However, both calcineurin inhibitors are associated with significant adverse effects including nephrotoxicity, hypertension, glucose intolerance, and hyperlipidemia that can negatively impact both graft and patient survival.[4-6]

Calcineurin Inhibitor Avoidance or Minimization

Several trials have been conducted aiming to avoid, minimize, withdraw, or convert calcineurin inhibitors. Initial calcineurin inhibitor avoidance as well as cyclosporine withdrawal in the setting of mycophenolate mofetil and corticosteroids has been associated with higher rates of acute rejection.[31-33] Other immunosuppressive agents utilized in place of the calcineurin inhibitor in attempt to preserve renal function have included the mammalian target of rapamycin (mTOR) inhibitors, sirolimus and everolimus, as well as the most recently approved maintenance immunosuppressive agent, belatacept.

When comparing de novo tacrolimus to sirolimus in the setting of rabbit ATG induction, mycophenolate mofetil, and corticosteroids; while patient survival, graft survival, and acute rejection rates were similar, there was no difference in mean glomerular filtration rate (GFR) as measured by iothalamate clearance between groups at 1 or 2 years post-transplantation.[34] In addition, 38% of patients in the sirolimus group discontinued the medication with the most common reasons including wound healing and pulmonary complications.[34] In the ELITE-symphony study, kidney transplant patients were randomly assigned in a 1:1:1:1 ratio to 1 of 4 treatment groups: standard-dose cyclosporine, low-dose cyclosporine, low-dose tacrolimus, or low-dose sirolimus, in combination with mycophenolate mofetil and corticosteroids. At 1-year post-transplantation, the mean calculated GFR (cGFR) was significantly higher, rate of biopsy proven acute rejection was significantly lower, and allograft survival was significantly higher in the low-dose tacrolimus group.[35] Importantly, treatment failure, defined as the use of additional immunosuppressive medication, the discontinuation of any study medication for >14 consecutive days or >30 cumulative days, allograft loss, or death, was highest in the low-dose sirolimus group at 35.8% ($p < 0.001$).[35] Overall, calcineurin inhibitor avoidance has not been widely adapted due to high rates of withdrawal, medication-related adverse effects, and/or lack of efficacy.

Many studies have been conducted attempting to convert calcineurin inhibitors to mTOR inhibitors; however, these strategies have had mixed results.[36–40] In the CONVERT trial, kidney transplant patients maintained on cyclosporine or tacrolimus were randomized to either continue calcineurin inhibitor therapy or to convert to sirolimus. In the primary intent-to-treat analysis, mean cGFR at 12 and 24 months was not significantly different between groups, however in a subgroup analysis in patients with baseline GFR >40 mL/min who remained on assigned therapy, mean cGFR was significantly higher after sirolimus conversion. However, significantly more patients that underwent sirolimus conversion discontinued treatment, and in patients with a baseline GFR of 20–40 mL/min, enrollment was halted early due to a higher incidence of acute rejection, graft loss, or death in the sirolimus conversion group. More treatment emergent adverse events including infection as well as higher median urinary protein-to-creatinine ratios postconversion occurred in the sirolimus group, although malignancy rates were significantly lower.[36] In the Spare-the-Nephron trial, compared to those maintained on calcineurin inhibitor-based therapy, patients converted to sirolimus had a significantly greater improvement in measured GFR at 1 year; however, change in GFR did not significantly differ between groups at 2 years.[37] Overall, conversion from calcineurin inhibitors to mTOR inhibitors does not appear to consistently offer a sustained benefit in renal function and is more commonly associated with treatment discontinuation.

These agents do have a unique side effect profile and are an alternative in patients intolerant to calcineurin inhibitors and/or patients that develop or are at high risk for malignancies including post-transplant skin cancers, perhaps with a particular niche in such circumstances given their antineoplastic effects.[41] While mTOR inhibitors were increasingly utilized in kidney transplant patients from 2000 to 2004, incidence peaked in 2003 at 18% and then subsequently decreased. As of 2010, only 5.9% of patients are maintained on these agents at 1-year post-transplantation.[7]

Belatacept, a selective T-cell costimulation blocker approved by the FDA in 2011, is an additional alternative to calcineurin inhibitor-based immunosuppressive therapy and is approved for use in adult kidney transplantation in combination with basiliximab induction, mycophenolate mofetil, and corticosteroids. It acts by blocking the CD28 mediated costimulation of T lymphocytes by binding to CD80 and CD86 on antigen-presenting cells, inhibiting T lymphocyte activation and proliferation.[42] In addition to its novel mechanism of action, belatacept differs from other available maintenance immunosuppressive agents in terms of route of administration, since it can only be given intravenously. In the BENEFIT and BENEFIT-EXT phase III studies, two belatacept-based regimens [more intensive (MI) and less intensive (LI) dosing] were compared to a cyclosporine (CsA)-based regimen in kidney transplant recipients of living or standard criteria donors and extended criteria donors, respectively.[43-46] In the BENEFIT study, renal function was superior in both belatacept-based dosing regimens compared to the cyclosporine regimen as defined by a coprimary composite renal impairment endpoint; percent of patients exhibiting a measured GFR <60 mL/min/1.73 m^2 at month 12 or a decrease in measured GFR ≥10 mL/min/1.73 m^2 from months 3 through 12 (MI=55%, LI=54%, CsA=78%; $p<0.0001$).[43] At 3 years, although measured GFR was not assessed, renal function remained better in the belatacept groups with a consistently higher mean cGFR, using the modification of diet in renal disease (MDRD) equation, over time compared to the cyclosporine group with a 15–21 mL/min/1.73 m^2 difference in mean cGFR observed.[45] In the BENEFIT-EXT study, at 12 months, fewer patients reached the composite renal impairment endpoint in the belatacept groups and this was statistically significant for the MI belatacept regimen and approached statistical significance for the LI belatacept regimen as compared to cyclosporine [MI=71%, LI=77%, CsA=85%; $p=0.002$ (MI vs CsA), $p=0.06$ (LI vs CsA)].[44] By year 3, mean cGFR was higher in the belatacept groups as compared to the cyclosporine-treated patients, with a mean estimated difference of 11 mL/min/1.73 m^2.[46] While the incidence of acute rejection at 12 months in the BENEFIT-EXT study was similar in the belatacept groups as compared to the cyclosporine group, it was higher in the belatacept groups in the BENEFIT study (MI=22%, LI=17%, CsA=7%).[43,44] In both studies, belatacept was associated with similar 1-year and 3-year patient and graft survival as compared to cyclosporine but notably more cases of PTLD; five in each study were observed with belatacept-based regimens within 3 years.[43–46]

The rate of PTLD was ninefold higher in patients who were Epstein–Barr virus (EBV) seronegative or with unknown serostatus compared to those who were EBV seropositive and due to this, belatacept is contraindicated for use in such patients.[47] Because there appeared to be no additional efficacy gained using the MI belatacept dosing regimen, the LI dosing regimen was chosen for the FDA approved regimen and higher than the recommended doses or more frequent dosing of belatacept are not recommended since total immunosuppression burden is a risk factor for PTLD. Frequency of infections was similar between belatacept and cyclosporine groups in trials with the exception of more tuberculosis in belatacept-treated patients.[45,46] There were also two fatal cases of progressive multifocal leukoencephalopathy (PML) in patients treated with belatacept, although none with the recommended dosing regimen.[47] An FDA mandated risk evaluation and mitigation strategy (REMS) has been established for belatacept to inform providers and patients of the increased risk of PTLD and PML in order to ensure that the benefits of the drug, including improvement in renal function as compared to cyclosporine-based therapy, outweigh these risks. Longer-term data are needed to further evaluate the safety profile of belatacept and associated risks.

Additional areas of investigation have included two phase II studies in kidney transplant recipients: an evaluation of belatacept-based, corticosteroid avoidance regimens and switching from calcineurin inhibitor-based regimens to a belatacept-based regimen. A small 12-month exploratory trial was conducted utilizing rabbit ATG induction and MI belatacept in combination with either sirolimus or mycophenolate mofetil and early CSWD after 4 days with a comparator group receiving tacrolimus and mycophenolate mofetil. Both belatacept groups experiences a relatively low incidence of acute rejection at 12 months comparable or better than previous trials utilizing calcineurin inhibitor avoidance and/or corticosteroid avoidance/withdrawal [belatacept/MMF=15% (5/33), belatacept/SRL=4% (1/26), tacrolimus/MMF=3% (1/30)]. Renal function was better in belatacept groups based on mean cGFR and no cases of PTLD or PML occurred.[48] A larger multicenter randomized clinical trial is currently ongoing and assessing belatacept with mycophenolate and early CSWD in the setting of alemtuzumab or rabbit ATG induction (www.clinicaltrials.gov). A randomized study investigated the safety and efficacy of switching stable kidney transplant patients, 6–36 month post-transplant, from maintenance calcineurin inhibitor therapy (either cyclosporine or tacrolimus) to a belatacept-based regimen. At 12 months, mean cGFR was slightly higher in the belatacept group as compared calcineurin inhibitor therapy continuation (60.5 mL/min/1.73 m^2 with an increase in 7 mL/min from baseline vs 56.5 mL/min/1.73 m^2 with an increase in 2.1 mL/min from baseline in the CNI group) although the study was not adequately powered to assess the statistical significance of the change from baseline in cGFR between the groups. Additionally, six patients (7.1%) switched to belatacept experienced acute rejection.[49] While this strategy may be feasible with a small risk of acute rejection, additional studies with adequate power need to be conducted to assess if a significant improvement in renal function is observed.

Overall, belatacept represents a novel maintenance immunosuppressive agent and an alternative to calcineurin inhibitor therapy in EBV seropositive kidney transplant patients; although longer-term follow-up and additional data are needed to determine its role and benefit vs risk profile including larger, randomized controlled comparative trials with tacrolimus-based maintenance immunosuppression.

Corticosteroid Minimization

While corticosteroids have been a cornerstone of immunosuppressive therapy in solid organ transplantation since the 1960s, they also have multiple side effects including hypertension, glucose intolerance, hyperlipidemia, and weight gain which can contribute to associated cardiovascular morbidity and mortality. Given this adverse effect profile, several studies over the past two decades have been conducted to assess the impact of CSWD or avoidance.[50-57] In early studies, CSWD attempted later post-transplant (≥3 months) and in the setting of cyclosporine-based maintenance immunosuppression was associated with significantly higher rates of acute rejection.[50,51] Additionally, in an early multicenter, randomized double-blind clinical trial, in patients maintained on cyclosporine and prednisone, long-term graft survival (5 years) was significantly lower in patients that were withdrawn from prednisone 3 months post-transplant compared to those maintained on prednisone. However, because temporary recourse to steroid therapy was allowed after randomization and occurred in over half of patients, these data are difficult to interpret.[50] Since the advent of more potent induction immunosuppression and maintenance therapy including tacrolimus and mycophenolate mofetil as well as advances in detection and characterization of anti-HLA antibodies to better assess immunological risk, CSWD and avoidance studies have had more encouraging results. Woodle et al. conducted a prospective, randomized, double-blind, placebo-controlled multicenter trial comparing early CSWD at 7 days with long-term low-dose corticosteroid therapy after kidney transplantation in the setting of concomitant tacrolimus and mycophenolate mofetil maintenance immunosuppression. Notably, patients with a current PRA ≥25% and/or peak PRA ≥50% as well as those with delayed graft function were excluded.

At 5 years, graft survival, patient survival, renal function, and incidence of moderate/severe acute rejection were similar between groups, although biopsy proven acute rejection approached statistical significance with a higher incidence in the CSWD group (17.8% vs 10.8%; p=0.058).[58] In terms of cardiovascular endpoints, there was no difference between groups in blood pressure, HDL cholesterol, LDL cholesterol, or incidence of new onset diabetes after transplant (NODAT), although there were statistically significant improvements in triglycerides, significantly less patients with NODAT requiring insulin therapy, and less weight gain from baseline in the CSWD group.[52] Corticosteroid avoidance and withdrawal in kidney transplantation continues to increase. In 1998, only 4.5% of kidney transplant recipients were discharged after kidney transplant without corticosteroids; however by 2011, 33.8% of patients were discharged on steroid-free maintenance immunosuppression.[7] Early CSWD, particularly in the setting of induction therapy and more potent maintenance immunosuppressive therapy including tacrolimus and mycophenolate, appears to be an effective and reasonable immunosuppressive strategy in select kidney transplant recipients that are not sensitized to preserve renal function in the intermediate term although longer-term data are needed.

Overall, maintenance immunosuppressive therapy has greatly evolved, and although calcineurin inhibitor based therapy with tacrolimus, mycophenolate +/- corticosteroids continues to be the standard and most commonly utilized regimen facilitating low rates of acute rejection, associated medication-related toxicities continue to contribute to morbidity and mortality. Maintenance immunosuppressive agents with different toxicity profiles offer alternatives to the individual patient allowing for more choice and personalization of immunosuppressive therapy.

ADDITIONAL CONSIDERATIONS IN PERSONALIZING IMMUNOSUPPRESSION

Several available immunosuppressive agents including tacrolimus, cyclosporine, sirolimus, and everolimus have a narrow therapeutic index due to significant interpatient and intrapatient variability. This variability can be due to pre-existing factors including activity and associated genetic polymorphisms of cytochrome P450 3A enzymes and the transport protein p-glycoprotein, clinical status (time after transplant, liver function, gut function), and presence of concomitant medications that inhibit or induce CYP 450 3A enzymes and/or p-glycoprotein. Additionally, over time as survival has improved, kidney transplant patients have an increasing number of comorbidities including seizure disorders, HIV, and hepatitis C for which multiple drug-drug interactions often exist with associated pharmacotherapy and transplant-related medications. Because of these factors, close therapeutic drug monitoring of these agents and associated individualization of dosing is an important component of post-transplant care. While there are several potential pharmacodynamic and pharmacokinetic drug interactions with immunosuppressive agents, those with drug metabolizing enzymes (i.e. CYP 450 enzymes) and drug transporter systems (i.e. p-glycoprotein) are frequently encountered. Tacrolimus, cyclosporine, sirolimus, and everolimus are all CYP3A substrates; thus if a concomitant medication is instituted that inhibits CYP3A, increased blood concentrations of the immunosuppressive agent can result. Conversely, medications that are inducers of CYP3A can lead to decreased blood concentrations of these immunosuppressive agents. Common CYP3A inhibitors and inducers are listed in Table 11.2. The severity of the drug-drug interactions are variable, and it is important to consult recommendations for each individual interaction in question for optimal management in the individual patient.

The pharmacogenomics of organ transplantation is an evolving field with several gene polymorphisms under investigation including those of CYP3A5, ABCB1, IMPDH1 and IMPDH2, and cytokines and growth factors.[58,59] Although gene expression assays are not widely available, in the future clinical pharmacogenomics could become a routine part of transplant clinical practice that allows for more individualization and targeted immunosuppressive agent dosing.

CONCLUSION

Kidney transplantation has greatly evolved and has seen many advances in immunosuppressive therapy, with an increasing number of immunosuppressive agents available for use in various combinations allowing for more choice and personalization of immunosuppressive therapy. Therapeutic developments have led to dramatically improved outcomes including lower acute kidney allograft rejection rates and improved allograft and patient survival. While maximizing efficacy and minimizing toxicity of immunosuppressive therapy continues to be a delicate balancing act, maintenance immunosuppression minimization strategies and targeted immune therapy continue to advance the transplant immunosuppression field. Emerging maintenance immunosuppressive agents that are void of nephrotoxic effects may lead to improvements in renal function as compared with the current standard of calcineurin inhibitor-based therapy. However, a one size fits all approach for any immunosuppressive strategy may not be best suited to the individual patient and ultimately patient-specific factors must be considered when designing the immunosuppressive regimen.

REFERENCES

1. Lamb KE, Lodhi S, Meier-Kriesche HU. Long-term renal allograft survival in the United State: a critical reappraisal. Am J Transplant. 2011;11:450-62.
2. Chapman JR, O'Connell PJ, Nankivell BJ. Chronic renal allograft dysfunction. J Am Soc Nephrol. 2005;16:3015-26.
3. Collins AJ, Foley RN, Herzog C, et al. US Renal Data System 2012 Annual Data Report. Am J Kidney Dis. 2013;61(1 Suppl 1):A7, e283-94.
4. Kirk AD, Mannon RD, Swanson SJ, et al. Strategies for minimizing immunosuppression in kidney transplantation. Transpl Int. 2005;18:2-14.
5. Yang H. Maintenance immunosuppression regimens: conversion, minimization, withdrawal, and avoidance. Am J Kidney Dis. 2006;47:S37-51.
6. Kramer BK, Zulke C, Kammerl MC, et al. Cardiovascular risk factors and estimated risk for CAD in a randomized trial comparing calcineurin inhibitors in renal transplantation. Am J Transplant. 2003;3:982-7.
7. Organ Procurement and Transplantation Network (OPTN) and Scientific Registry of Transplant Recipients (SRTR). OPTN/SRTR 2011 Annual Data Report. Rockville, MD: Department of Health and Human Services, Health Resources and Services Administration, Healthcare Systems Bureau, Division of Transplantation; 2011.
8. Brennan DC, Flavin K, Lowell JA, et al. A randomized, double-blinded comparison of Thymoglobulin versus ATGAM for induction immunosuppressive therapy in adult renal transplant recipients. Transplantation. 1999;67:1011-8.
9. Thymoglobulin® [package insert]. Cambridge, MA: Genzyme Corporation; 2008.
10. Bonnefoy-Berard N, Revillard JP. Mechanisms of immunosuppression induced by antithymocyte globulins and OKT3. J Heart Lung Transplant. 1996;15:435-42.
11. Préville X, Flacher M, LeMauff B, et al. Mechanisms involved in antithymocyte globulin immunosuppressive activity in a nonhuman primate model. Transplantation. 2001;15:460-8.
12. Berard JL, Velez RL, Freeman RB, et al. A review of interleukin-2 receptor antagonists in solid organ transplantation. Pharmacotherapy. 1999;19:1127-37.
13. Nashan B, Moore R, Amlot P, et al. Randomised trial of basiliximab versus placebo for control of acute cellular rejection in renal allograft recipients. CHIB 201 International Study Group. Lancet. 1997;350:1193-8.
14. Kahan BD, Rajagopalan PR, Hall M, et al. Reduction of the occurrence of acute cellular rejection among renal allograft recipients treated with basiliximab, a chimeric anti-interleukin-2-receptor monoclonal antibody. United States Simulect Renal Study Group. Transplantation. 1999;67:276-84.
15. Sollinger H, Kaplan B, Pescovitz MD, et al. Basiliximab versus antithymocyte globulin for prevention of acute renal allograft rejection. Transplantation. 2001;72:1915-9.
16. Brennan DC, Daller JA, Lake KD, et al. Rabbit antithymocyte globulin versus basiliximab in renal transplantation. N Engl J Med. 2006;355:1967-77.
17. Calne R, Friend P, Moffatt S, et al. Prope tolerance, perioperative campath 1H, and low-dose cyclosporin monotherapy in renal allograft recipients. Lancet. 1998;351:1701-2.
18. Kirk AD, Hale DA, Mannon RB, et al. Results from a human renal allograft tolerance trial evaluating the humanized CD52-specific monoclonal antibody alemtuzumab (CAMPATH-1H). Transplantation. 2003;76:120-9.
19. Genzyme Corporation. US Campath distribution program [internet]. 2012 [cited 2013 Nov 13]. Available from http://www.campath.com.

20. Watson CJ, Bradley JA, Friend PJ, et al. Alemtuzumab (CAMPATH 1H) induction therapy in cadaveric kidney transplantation - efficacy and safety at five years. Am J Transplant. 2005;5:1347-53.
21. Kaufman DB, Leventhal JR, Axelrod D, et al. Alemtuzumab induction and prednisone-free maintenance immunotherapy in kidney transplantation: comparison with basiliximab induction - long-term results. Am J Transplant. 2005;5:2539-48.
22. Tan HP, Kaczorowski DJ, Basu A, et al. Living donor renal transplantation using alemtuzumab induction and tacrolimus monotherapy. Am J Transplant. 2006;6:2409-17.
23. Ciancio G, Burke GW, Gaynor JJ, et al. A randomized trial of three renal transplant induction antibodies: early comparison of tacrolimus, mycophenolate mofetil, and steroid dosing, and newer immune-monitoring. Transplantation. 2005;80:457-65.
24. Hanaway MJ, Woodle ES, Mulgaonkar S, et al. Alemtuzumab induction in renal transplantation. N Engl J Med. 2011;364:1909-19.
25. Kirk AD, Cherikh WS, Ring M, et al. Dissociation of depletional induction and posttransplant lymphoproliferative disease in kidney recipients treated with alemtuzumab. Am J Transplant. 2007;7:2619-25.
26. Vincenti F, Laskow DA, Neylan JF, et al. One-year follow-up of an open-label trial of FK506 for primary kidney transplantation. A report of the U.S. Multicenter FK506 Kidney Transplant Group. Transplantation. 1996;61:1576-81.
27. Pirsch JD, Miller J, Deierhoi MH, et al. A comparison of tacrolimus (FK506) and cyclosporine for immunosuppression after cadaveric renal transplantation. FK506 Kidney Transplant Study Group. Transplantation. 1997;63:977-83.
28. Mayer AD, Dmitrewski J, Squifflet JP, et al. Multicenter randomized trial comparing tacrolimus (FK506) and cyclosporine in the prevention of renal allograft rejection: a report of the European Tacrolimus Multicenter Renal Study Group. Transplantation. 1997;64:436-43.
29. Abouljoud MS, Kumar MS, Brayman KL, et al. Neoral rescue therapy in transplant patients with intolerance to tacrolimus. Clin Transplant. 2002;16:168-72.
30. Oberholzer J, Thielke J, Hatipoglu B, et al. Immediate conversion from tacrolimus to cyclosporine in the treatment of posttransplantation diabetes mellitus. Transplant Proc. 2005;37:999-1000.
31. Vincenti F, Ramos E, Brattstrom C, et al. Multicenter trial exploring calcineurin inhibitors avoidance in renal transplantation. Transplantation. 2001;71:1282-87.
32. Ekberg H, Grinyó J, Nashan B, et al. Cyclosporine sparing with mycophenolate mofetil, daclizumab and corticosteroids in renal allograft recipients: the CAESAR Study. Am J Transplant. 2007;7:560-70.
33. Abramowicz D, Del Carmen Rial M, Vitko S, et al. Cyclosporine withdrawal from a mycophenolate mofetil-containing immunosuppressive regimen: results of a five-year, prospective, randomized study. J Am Soc Nephrol. 2005;16:2234-40.
34. Larson TS, Dean PG, Stegall MD, et al. Complete avoidance of calcineurin inhibitors in renal transplantation: a randomized trial comparing sirolimus and tacrolimus. Am J Transplant. 2006;6:514-22.
35. Ekberg H, Tedesco-Silva H, Demirbas A, et al. Reduced exposure to calcineurin inhibitors in renal transplantation. N Engl J Med. 2007;357:2562-75.
36. Schena FP, Pascoe MD, Alberu J, et al. Conversion from calcineurin inhibitors to sirolimus maintenance therapy in renal allograft recipients: 24-month efficacy and safety results from the CONVERT trial. Transplantation. 2009;87:233-42.

37. Weir MR, Mulgaonkar S, Chan L, et al. Mycophenolate mofetil-based immunosuppression with sirolimus in renal transplantation: a randomized, controlled Spare-the-Nephron trial. Kidney Int. 2011;79:897-907.
38. Holdaas H, Rostaing L, Serón D, et al. Conversion of long-term kidney transplant recipients from calcineurin inhibitor therapy to everolimus: a randomized, multicenter, 24-month study. Transplantation. 2011;92:410-18.
39. Budde K, Becker T, Arns W, et al. Everolimus-based, calcineurin-inhibitor-free regimen in recipients of de-novo kidney transplants: an open-label, randomised, controlled trial. Lancet. 2011;377:837-47.
40. Heilman RL, Younan K, Wadei HM, et al. Results of a prospective randomized trial of sirolimus conversion in kidney transplant recipients on early corticosteroid withdrawal. Transplantation. 2011;92:767-73.
41. Campbell SB, Walker R, Tai SS, et al. Randomized controlled trial of sirolimus for renal transplant recipients at high risk for nonmelanoma skin cancer. Am J Transplant. 2012;12:1146-56.
42. Vincenti F, Larsen C, Durrbach A, et al. Costimulation blockade with belatacept in renal transplantation. N Engl J Med. 2005;353:770-81.
43. Vincenti F, Charpentier B, Vanrenterghem Y, et al. A phase III study of belatacept-based immunosuppression regimens versus cyclosporine in renal transplant recipients (BENEFIT study). Am J Transplant. 2010;10:535-46.
44. Durrbach A, Pestana JM, Pearson T, et al. A phase III study of belatacept versus cyclosporine in kidney transplants from extended criteria donors (BENEFIT-EXT Study). Am J Transplant. 2010;10:547-57.
45. Vincenti F, Larsen CP, Alberu J, et al. Three-year outcomes from BENEFIT, a randomized, active-controlled, parallel-group study in adult kidney transplant recipients. Am J Transplant. 2012;12:210-7.
46. Pestana JO, Grinyo JM, Vanrenterghem Y, et al. Three-year outcomes from BENEFIT-EXT: a phase III study of belatacept versus cyclosporine in recipients of extended criteria donor kidneys. Am J Transplant. 2012;12:630-39.
47. Nulojix [package insert]. Princeton, NJ: Bristol-Myers Squibb Company; 2011.
48. Ferguson R, Grinyo J, Vincenti F, et al. Immunosuppression with belatacept-based, corticosteroid-avoiding regimens in de novo kidney transplant recipients. Am J Transplant. 2011;11:66-76.
49. Rostaing L, Massari P, Garcia VD, et al. Switching from calcineurin inhibitor-based regimens to a belatacept-based regimen in renal transplant recipients: a randomized phase II study. Clin J Am Soc Nephrol. 2011;6:430-39.
50. Sinclair NR. Low-dose steroid therapy in cyclosporine-treated renal transplant recipients with well-functioning grafts. The Canadian Multicentre Transplant Study Group. CMAJ. 1992;147:645-57.
51. Vanrenterghem Y, Lebranchu Y, Hené R, et al. Double-blind comparison of two corticosteroid regimens plus mycophenolate mofetil and cyclosporine for prevention of acute renal allograft rejection. Transplantation. 2000;70:1352-59.
52. Woodle ES, First MR, Pirsch J, et al. A prospective, randomized, double-blind, placebo-controlled multicenter trial comparing early (7 day) corticosteroid cessation versus long-term, low-dose corticosteroid therapy. Ann Surg. 2008; 248(4):564-77.
53. Ratcliffe PJ, Dudley CR, Higgins RM, et al. Randomised controlled trial of steroid withdrawal in renal transplant recipients receiving triple immunosuppression. Lancet. 1996;348:643-8.

54. Schulak JA, Mayes JT, Moritz CE, et al. A prospective randomized trial of prednisone versus no prednisone maintenance therapy in cyclosporine-treated and azathioprine-treated renal transplant patients. Transplantation. 1990;49:327-32.
55. Vanrenterghem Y, van Hooff JP, Squifflet JP, et al. Minimization of immunosuppressive therapy after renal transplantation: results of a randomized trial. Am J Transplant. 2005;5:87-95.
56. Woodle ES, Peddi VR, Tomlanovich S, et al. A prospective, randomized, multicenter study evaluating early corticosteroid withdrawal with Thymoglobulin in living-donor kidney transplantation. Clin Transplant. 2010;24:73-83.
57. Kramer BK, Klinger M, Vitko S, et al. Tacrolimus-based, steroid-free regimens in renal transplantation: 3-year follow-up of the ATLAS trial. Transplantation. 2012;94:492-8.
58. MacPhee IA. Use of pharmacogenetics to optimize immunosuppressive therapy. Ther Drug Monit. 2010;32:261-4.
59. Burckart GJ, Amur S. Update on the clinical pharmacogenomics of organ transplantation. Pharmacogenomics. 2010;11:227-36.

Index

Page numbers followed by *f* refer to figure and *t* refer to table

H

I

K

L

M

N